THE *OTHER*
MID-LIFE CRISIS

Everything You Need to Know About
Wills, Hospitals, Life-and-Death
Decisions and Final Matters
(but were never taught)

Adeline Rosemire

▲ Meridian Publishing, Inc.
San Jose, California

This book contains only general information that may be proper for use in simple transactions and in no way acts, or is intended to act, as a substitute for the advice of an attorney. The publisher does not make any warranty, either express or implied, about the validity of any provision or the suitability of information found in this book as to any specific transaction.

Dedication

In honor of my father,
Henry M. Azevedo, Jr. (1917 - 1991)
and my brother,
Alvin H. Azevedo (1956 - 1993)

Acknowledgments

Special thanks to my husband, and editor, Mike (now-don't-take-this-personally) Rosemire.

For sharing their professional insights and real-life experiences, I would like to thank the following for contributing immeasurably to this book:

Judy Wilson Lynn

Gloria E. Salas

Dorothy Sanches

Gary E. M. Smith, O.D.

Jean P. Sukovez

Ann Thompson

Patricia Tobin, Esq.

Introduction

It takes a long time to learn certain things about life. Years. This book represents the short-course approach to a segment of life that most people will encounter when they can least cope. It's about life, death, and the place in between. This book will save you time and provide you with information that took other people years to learn.

I wrote this book to help people avoid what my family and I went through when my father suffered a massive stroke. He was almost completely paralyzed and spent 6 years in a skilled nursing facility until his death. My mother was with him every day. My brother died from complications of Hodgkin's Disease at the age of 37. He read the first draft of this book; sadly, his recent death put this book to the ultimate test. This book doesn't have all the answers, but I hope that it will help you get through whatever you might face in life.

This book is not intended to be used as legal or medical advice or to endorse any product or service. It is meant to serve as a general informational resource and guide, not as a substitute for professional help.

Contents

20 Fast Facts

Here is 5 minutes of reading that will put you years ahead of almost everyone else in the game of life. In other words, you'll be better prepared after reading this list.

- Find out now exactly how much coverage your spouse has in life insurance. It should be 5-6 times their annual salary if you have children and no other means of financial support. If one spouse earns 60% of the household income, that spouse should carry 60% of the life insurance.
- Check the accuracy of your future Social Security benefits by calling (800) 234-5772 and requesting Form SSA-7004-PC. A few weeks after returning the completed form, you will receive a Personal Earnings and Benefits Estimate Statement. Check it carefully for errors. Any discrepancies could rob you of rightful benefits.
- When a parent becomes destitute, the so-called 'poor laws' in many states require children to pay the parent's bills and reimburse the state for any support it provides.
- Losing a spouse translates into 200-300 hours of tears. Such a 'healing timetable' can take one to two years or more.
- Airlines and some hotels offer emergency and medical emergency rates. You must specifically ask about them.
- Most banks can waive early withdrawal penalties from CDs in an emergency.
- If you have a death certificate, you have the right to open the deceased's safe deposit box. Better yet, have your name added so that you may have access during an emergency.
- The Red Cross can help if a death occurs out of state or out of the country.
- For closed caskets, a liner isn't necessary or required.
- Keep a 5"x 7" spiral notebook with you. After the death of someone close to them, many people discover they don't have their usual ability to recall conversations and past decisions.
- Don't make a big financial mistake by neglecting to have assets professionally appraised promptly after a death. You'll need this information for tax purposes later.

- Making major decisions too quickly is another common error. People need time to recover. Example: Leave the proceeds of a life insurance policy with the insurance company so that it earns interest. Or simply put the money in a money-market fund while you gather information and figure out what you need to live on.

- If you are handling an estate, to save time and add convenience, make a change of address at the post office so that you will receive all mail pertaining to the estate.

- Obtain a file cabinet. And get ready for a mountain of paperwork. In one drawer put everything that relates to the decedent: pension, Social Security information, etc. In another drawer put information that relates to you: bank accounts, current bills, etc. Keep the estate-related files separate.

- Use manila file folders and accountants' columnar paper to keep track of medical bills. Headings: Provider, date of service, amount of bill, received by insurance, insurance paid amount & date, secondary insurance paid amount & date, balance, date balance paid and check number.

- To avoid dunning notices when handling an estate, gather bills that the decedent paid in the last 3 months. You can either arrive at an average monthly payment, or make a nominal payment on each account to avoid threats of turned off utilities, etc. You can also write and include a 'form letter' to explain the situation.

- If you are handling an estate and you can't locate information regarding the decedent's life insurance, go through his or her cancelled checks (at least 12 months). You will probably find a check made out to the life insurance company. If not, call The American Council of Life Insurance, (800) 942-4242, and ask about their free Policy Search service.

- Change traditions. Have holiday dinners at a different home this year. Unfortunately, if you try to make things as they were, it will make the absence of your spouse, child or friend more pronounced.

- To decrease stress, make decisions and preparations ahead of time to give you a sense of control over your life.

• Here's a useful glossary:

Advance directives—a generic term for legal documents (such as health-care powers of attorney and living wills) that state a person's medical treatment preferences

Annuities-arrangements with insurance companies and other financial institutions, under which money is transferred from the owner in return for a promise to make steady payments of income

Attorney in fact—the person you choose to make decisions on your behalf

Conservatee or ward— person being protected

Conservator— a person directed to handle only financial matters

Disposition— the manner in which a body is disposed of (ground burial, cremation, donation, or entombment)

Durable power of attorney— a document that legally empowers a person to perform a task for you. It stays in effect even after the incapacity of the principal (person who granted the power of attorney).

Executor/Executress/Administrator— a person who wraps up your affairs after your death

Fiduciary— a person who assumes responsibility for another person's financial affairs

Guardian— a person who handles only personal, not financial, decisions

Intestate— dying without a will

Ombudsman— an independent person who can investigate and resolve complaints made by residents of medical facilities

Power of attorney— a legal document that empowers someone to perform a task as long as the principal is capable

Probate— the legal procedure which leads to an estate's final distribution

Principal— person conferring power

Trust—a contract empowering someone to manage money or property

Trustee—the manager of a trust

Chapter 1

Paperwork
It only takes 5 steps to get your 'legal life' in good shape

"Estates should be left to loved ones, not attorneys." — Walter Heiden

"You own stuff. You will die. Someone will get your stuff." — Jane Bryant Quinn

"I think it's time to think about writing a will." — An 84-year-old woman telling her 87-year-old husband of her plans.

Important

A simple do-it-yourself will can cost as little as $6.95, the price of a paperback. If a will is prepared by a professional, it can cost up to $400 an hour. Make sure financial paperwork is in order *before* a crisis hits. It can save you and your family thousands of dollars later.

The downside of not being prepared:
• years of legal entanglement for survivors
• potentially unpleasant family dynamics
• financial loss
• lots of stress

Step one: Prepare a will

Do it yourself, or have a friend recommend a lawyer. Ask the lawyer about fees and his or her specialty. Set up an appointment. Take with you a list of the names and addresses of the people you want included in your will. Determine what sort of burial and/or service you want, if any. Appoint an executor; this is the person who will carry out the wishes listed in your will. Make sure your executor has a copy of your will. Many people have detailed funeral instructions in their will; but, by the time the will is read, the funeral is long over.

Writing a will can maintain independence and ensure that personal wishes are respected. Most people want to know what would happen if they were to die before their kids reach 18.

People are relieved to learn they can appoint a personal guardian with a simple will.

Don't assume that an estate will go directly to a spouse or children. For instance, depending upon the state, a surviving spouse may receive 50% of the estate and the decedent's parents may receive 50%.

Where there's a will, there's a way to cut taxes via trust funds and charitable trusts. For the newest and most effective methods consult an attorney, certified public accountant, chartered life underwriter, trust officer, planned giving specialist or probate attorney.

Remember to:
• Update your will every 10 years or sooner.
• Revise your will if you move to a new state.
• Rework your will if there are any major changes in your family.

TIP: You can write your own will using the new computer applications available. *The Simple Will Book* by attorney Denis Clifford is also a good choice for do-it-yourselfers.

Step two: Prepare a living will

A living will is also called a Declaration to Physicians or a Directive to Physicians. This document, recognized by over 40 states, allows a physician to respect a patient's instruction to permit an imminent death to proceed naturally. Although living wills may not legally hold up in every state in the country, at least your wishes will be stated in writing. Living wills state a person's decision to refuse medical treatment, particularly artificial life support.

You don't need a lawyer to prepare a living will	You can find living will forms in many office supply/stationery stores. You can also obtain the forms free by sending a self-addressed stamped envelope to the Society for the Right to Die, 250 W. 57th St., New York, NY 10107. (212) 246-6973.
Keep a copy with your will	To avoid dissention, let everyone involved know about your decisions. Doctors, hospitals, nursing homes and family members can't honor a living will or power of attorney if they don't have a copy of it. Then again, some people don't ever want the 'plug pulled' and don't need this document.

Step three: Consider a durable power of attorney

Durable power of attorney forms are available in stationery stores, hospitals and some physicians' offices. These forms do not require the intervention of a lawyer; however, most people would feel most comfortable getting legal (and perhaps financial) advice before signing such significant documents. If you decide to use a professional to draft these documents, be sure to consult an attorney who specializes in estate matters. The fee typically ranges from $50-$150 for a 5-6 page document.

A *durable power of attorney* is a legal document that enables someone to handle your affairs if you become incapacitated.

A *durable power of attorney for health care* allows you to choose the person (a trusted relative and/or friend, not necessarily your lawyer) who will make health care decisions for you if you are unable to make them yourself.

Most states allow a *springing power of attorney*, a legal document that does not become effective until the principal becomes incapacitated.

Give a copy to the people you have asked to handle your affairs

Remember to give a copy to your selected attorney-in-fact and review the documents every few years. In some states, the directives expire several years from the date they are signed. Even if you don't complete these forms, you might consider writing down your wishes, or at least telling your physician, minister or appropriate family members.

Step four: Consider a living trust	If you are older or have considerable assets, a living trust can benefit you and your heirs, by: • providing for your living expenses and other benefits while you are alive • avoiding probate (an expensive and time-consuming process) • protecting a spouse from poverty • avoiding an expensive and intrusive conservatorship or guardianship (in which the court appoints a decision-maker for you) • preserving your privacy (the terms of a trust are private) A living trust allows you to choose who controls and manages your affairs. It usually takes effect immediately and deals with your financial affairs for the rest of your life and after your death. Some attorneys prepare stand-by trusts. An *inter vivos living trust* allows you to be both trustee and beneficiary. When one spouse dies or becomes incompetent, the other takes over. After both die, the living trust can specify a child, a relative, a friend or other entity to become the new trustee and new beneficiary. This will avoid probate costs and delays.
Not averting estate taxes is a mistake	Probate fees on even a small estate can add up to several thousand dollars. Probate fees on a $200,000 house can add up to $15,000.
Naming names	A trust specifies, among other things, beneficiaries and managers. You may wish to name a person to co-manage the trust with you for a test period to see how they would perform before they take full responsibility. Consider appointing co-trustees— a

professional and a relative— for the best of both sides: expert management and family sensibilities.

You sign the documents and then take steps to transfer the assets (such as home and bank accounts) into the trust. You will have the same control over your assets as before; however, the form of ownership will have changed.

Benefits   You will almost undoubtedly have saved money, retained control of your assets, and provided for your family's future needs, as well as your own. Remember, unless you make provisions, current tax rules provide that assets over $600,000 can be taxed at rates ranging from 37-55%. The first $600,000 passes along without any estate taxes ($1.2 million if you use a simple 'bypass' trust).

Important   While a living trust is an excellent estate planning device, it is not appropriate in all situations. Contact an attorney and/or an accountant for tax and estate planning issues. Trust and estate planning departments at banks also can manage investments for a fee. Scoundrels abound, so deal only with reputable people.

TIPS: For more information, send a postcard requesting *"Living Trusts & Wills"*, #D14535, to: AARP Fulfillment, 601 E. St., NW, Washington, DC 20049

For information about how to select an elder law attorney, send a SASE (self- addressed stamped envelope) to:
National Academy of Elder Law Attorneys
655 N. Alvernon Way, Suite 108
Tucson, Arizona 85711

Bonus points — or Step five

For the ultra-organized, you may wish to consolidate information, or its whereabouts, in an informal Letter of Instruction to those you love. This is also the best place to record your preferences and plans for disposition and funeral or memorial arrangements. The following brief statement written on a separate sheet of paper will eliminate any question of whether or not you wish to be cremated.

TO WHOM IT MAY CONCERN:

I, _____, wish to instruct those person or persons in charge of my remains to cremate my body and under no circumstances to provide for any embalming and burial, or either.

Date: _____

Signature: _____

Print name: _____

This is easier than it looks

Don't let the huge list that follows scare you; a lot of the items and documents won't pertain to everyone. The goal is to produce a guide to your important 'stuff'. This guide will be extremely helpful to someone if they need to step in for you to handle your affairs.

Keep a copy of List A and List B in your safe deposit box and give a copy to the person who will be handling your affairs. Be sure your executor/executress has the key and legal access to the box. Don't include your name or address on the list; this will protect you in case the lists are stolen or misplaced.

List A - Location of information and important items

Date: _____

Most people keep important information in several locations, such as a safe deposit box, a file cabinet or under a non-interest-bearing mattress. Below, note your locations. Example: Location 1 <u>Top drawer in chest of drawers located in master bedroom.</u>

(It is typical to have 3-8 locations.)

Location 1

_____

Location 2

_____

Location 3

_____

Location 4

_____

Location 5

_____

Location 6

_____

Location 7

_____

Location 8

_____

Location 9

_____

Location 10

_____

Location 11

_____

Location 12

_____

Notes:

List B - Important Items

There are two ways to do this step. The quickest way is to write the location number (from List A) next to the items found below on List B. *Example:* _2_ *address book.* (The address book is found in the second location listed.) See completed example on following page.

For people who want the information on one piece of paper, on List A you can write the separate items that can be found in their respective locations.
Example: Location 1: top drawer in the chest of drawers in the master bedroom—bank account books, checkbook, passport.

Don't whine. This should take you an hour, tops. You will have saved someone you love days, or maybe years, of work. And you will experience a sensation of relief and accomplishment. Promise.

____ address book

____ accountant's address and phone number

____ accounts receivable list (debts owed to you)

____ adoption papers

____ annulment papers

____ attorney's address & phone number

____ auto insurance policies

____ auto registration 'pink slip'

____ bank account numbers and bank addresses

____ baptismal certificate

____ household contents

____ household insurance

____ investments

____ jewelry and other items of intrinsic value

____ IRA and 401(k) agreements

____ keepsakes

____ Keogh agreement (self-employment retirement plan)

____ leases

____ life insurance policies

____ loans outstanding

____ marriage certificate(s)

____ Medicaid and Medicare cards and stickers

____ military service discharge and records (include 'C' number for older veterans)

____ manuscripts and original works of art not on display

____ mortgage papers

____ naturalization papers

____ pension agreements

____ post office box and key

____ power of attorney

____ pre-paid funeral plan (if any)

____ profit-sharing plans

____ railroad retirement documents

____ real estate records

____ record of assets/liabilities

____ registration papers for animals

____ safe deposit box key and bank addresss

____ savings account books

____ stockbroker account number

____ stockbroker statements

____ stock certificates

____ Social Security card and numbers of all family members

____ state and federal income tax returns from prior years

____ stock certificates

____ tax returns

____ trusts

____ uniform donor card (for organ donations)

____ warranties

____ will and location of original

____ Worker's compensation agreement

____ W-2 forms (current)

Samples of List A and List B

List A - Location of information and important items   Date: _____

Most people keep important information in several locations, such as a safe deposit box, a file cabinet or under a non-interest-bearing mattress. Below, note your locations. Example:
Location 1 <u>Top drawer in chest of drawers located in master bedroom.</u>

(It is typical to have 3-8 locations.)

Location 1
_____ *top drawer, chest of drawers, master bedroom*
Location 2
_____ *desk in guestroom, 2nd drawer*
Location 3
_____ *File cabinet in guest bedroom, top drawer*
Location 4
_____ *safe deposit box at Bank of the West on Hamilton*
Location 5
_____
Location 6
_____
Location 7
_____
Location 8
_____
Location 9
_____
Location 10
_____
Location 11
_____
Location 12
_____

Notes:

example of List A

List B - Important Items   Date: _____

There are two ways to do this step. The quickest way is to write the location number (from List A) next to the items found below on List B. *Example:* ___ *address book*. (The address book is found in the second location listed.) See completed example on following page.

For people who want the information on one piece of paper, on List A you can write the separate items that can be found in their respective locations.
Example: Location 1: top drawer in the chest of drawers in the master bedroom—bank account books, checkbook, passport.

Don't whine. This should take you an hour, tops. You will have saved someone you love days, or maybe years, of work. And you will experience a sensation of relief and accomplishment. Promise.

_1_ address book
_1_ accountant's address and phone number
_1_ accounts receivable list (debts owed to you)
_4_ adoption papers
_4_ annulment papers
_2_ attorney's address & phone number
_1_ auto insurance policies
_2_ auto registration 'pink slip'
_1_ bank account numbers and bank addresses
_2_ baptismal certificate
___ household contents
___ household insurance
_4_ investments
_4_ jewelry and other items of intrinsic value
___ IRA and 401(k) agreements
___ keepsakes
___ Keogh agreement (self-employment retirement plan)

_1_ leases
_1_ life insurance policies
___ loans outstanding
_1_ marriage certificate(s)
_3_ Medicaid and Medicare cards and stickers
_4_ military service discharge and records (include 'C' number for older veterans)
___ manuscripts and original works of art not on display
___ mortgage papers
_3_ naturalization papers
_3_ pension agreements
_1_ post office box and key
_1_ power of attorney
_2_ pre-paid funeral plan (if any)
_4_ profit-sharing plans
___ railroad retirement documents
___ real estate records
___ record of assets/liabilities
___ registration papers for animals
___ safe deposit box key and bank address

___ savings account books
___ stockbroker account number
___ stockbroker statements
___ stock certificates
___ Social Security card and numbers of all family members
_1_ state and federal income tax returns from prior years
_4_ stock certificates
___ tax returns
_3_ trusts
___ uniform donor card (for organ donations)
___ warranties
_1_ will and location of original
_1_ Worker's compensation agreement
_1_ W-2 forms (current)

example of List B

TIP: To put the information on your computer, try For the Record from Nolo Press, (510) 549-1976.

More bonus points: You should ask your parents three important questions *now*. Do this for your benefit, as well as for your parents' benefit. Most people don't like to talk about their own death. The good news is that you can avoid a crisis decision-making situation by asking only three questions; the bad news is that these are three of the most difficult questions you can ask yourself, your parents or your friends.

---

1. If you are incapacitated, who do you want to act in your behalf in terms of medical, financial and/or business considerations? (You can specify a different person for each category.)

_____

2. Do you want extreme measures taken to prolong your life? (Circle only one.)
      Yes   No

3. How do you want the details of your death handled? Choices:
burial (where?)_____ cremation_____ other_____
Services (type)_____
Special clothes (describe)_____
Organ donor? (Circle only one.)   Yes   No
Comments_____
Signature _____ Date _____

How to start It takes courage to ask these questions, but balancing needs is important. Suggest a meeting so your parents understand the seriousness of your intent.

To ease into the subjects of finances and personal records, treat these areas as part of an older person's rich past. For instance, ask them how long they've had their safe deposit box. Ask where the key is and what the box holds.

You can lead into the questions by using practical matters, such as asking, "I've been thinking about how someday you're going to be gone— is there anything you want me to know?" Asking your parents how they handled things with their parents is another good way to get a conversation started.

You can also send your parents articles about long-term-care insurance and housing options to pave the way for discussion. Spread out your questions over time, eventually you should have specific information as to:
• their choice of medical care
• how they expect to pay for long-term care if they need it
• whether they have durable powers of attorney
• the location of their important documents

An alternative to the previously-suggested approaches is to tell them that you are mailing something to them (the previous questionnaire) and ask that they return it to you completed and signed (enclose a self-addressed stamped envelope).

Encourage your parents to make up a personal affairs record while they are still capable of the task. Ask them about the items listed above. You'll need to be diplomatic and open-minded, especially if their style is different from yours.

The buddy system

Since most adults need to gather the same data, you can make this a joint effort, and this may be more palatable to your parents. What the heck— place a bet on who finishes first.

Or get your affairs in order first and tell your parents what you've learned. It may help them see that these arrangements are for everyone, not just older people.

Remember: if these approaches fail, at least you know you've met your responsibilities.

Will substitutes

Joint accounts are sometimes viewed as 'will substitutes'. When a joint tenant dies, the bank account automatically goes to the other joint tenant(s). Other methods include joint property status; revocable trusts; and 'Totten trusts' or 'payable on death' accounts, both of which direct the distribution of money to the person named by the principal.

More about estates

Some of the newest and most popular estate-planning techniques are family limited partnerships and grantor-retained income trusts (GRITs). Contact an attorney for details.

When someone dies, it is often necessary to evaluate real estate to determine a selling price. The established amount will serve as a base for:
• measuring the amount of estate taxes due
• distribution of assets
• placing a value for a buyout by a surviving partner
• establishing a framework within which executors or beneficiaries can make monetary decisions

For a free copy of the national directory of designated appraisers, write to: Society of Real Estate Appraisers, 645 N. Michigan Ave., Chicago, IL 60611.

TIP: Remember that most banks can only federally insure money up to $100,000 in a person's name, regardless of the number of accounts held at that bank.

Chapter 2

Insurance, Social Security, Medicare and Medicaid

Most older people are concerned that a prolonged illness may financially wipe them out. By thinking about health plans while you're healthy, you can take steps that will help prevent a calamity.

Insurance policies

**Ask yourself:
Will I need it?
Can I afford it?**

Consider the purchase of long-term-care (LTC) insurance by the age of 65, while it's still affordable. Policies usually pay a certain amount per day. Cost: $575-1,400 a year. The best policies are those with inflation protection riders. The Health Insurance Counseling and Advocacy Program (HICAP) can provide counseling and information: (800) 233-9045.

Other sources include:
• attorneys that specialize in elder care issues
• financial planners
• geriatric care managers
• competent/objective insurance representatives

Topping *Consumer Reports'* list of recommendations of insurance carriers that offer comprehensive policies (nursing-home and home-care) are:
• Atlantic & Pacific (800) 537-1688
• CNA (800) 327-2430
• Prudential-AARP (800) 523-5800

Note:

If permitted by your insurer, you may collect up to 95% of the face value of your life insurance policy while you are still alive. Check your state insurance department's rules on 'accelerated benefits' or ' viatical settlements'.

Medigap

Medicare supplemental insurance (Medigap) is available to supplement Part B of Medicare. If you can afford it, buy coverage

---

that will pay the entire unapproved portion of doctors' bills. Federal law requires that the 10 standard Medigap policies be uniform and standardized, so shop according to premiums and services offered by different insurance carriers. Premiums vary by as much as 70% for the same type of policy.

Low-cost providers include: Blue Cross, Blue Shield, Pyramid Life and Prudential. Also consider SecureHorizons, (800) 322-8877, which is accredited by the National Committee for Quality Assurance.

There are also new plans available that have no premium cost; they carry the provision that Medicare benefits will be assigned to the insurance company. Some plans also have prescription drug coverage.

Specialized policies   Hospital Confinement Indemnity coverage pays a fixed amount for each day you are in a hospital, up to a specified maximum number of days. This kind of coverage is generally not recommended because hospital stays are usually only 2-3 days; patients requiring longer recovery periods are usually sent to nursing homes.

A Specified Disease policy (not available in some states) provides benefits only if you become ill with a particular disease, such as cancer, and the benefits are usually limited to a certain dollar amount. These policies are typically not recommended because of their overall limitations.

In the future, more state governments will work with corporations—in partnership programs— to offer long-term-care group policies. Some current company plans offer coverage to parents and, in some cases, to in-laws of employees. California, Connecticut and Indiana will soon introduce additional 'partnership' programs.

Social Security

General information

The youngest starting age for a Social Security retirement pension is 62. However, Social Security coverage may be available for disabled wage earners or their dependents at a younger age. For people born before 1938, full retirement benefits are available at age 65. Ensure that registrations for Social Security and other programs are in order.

For estimates of your future retirement benefits, present survivors' benefits and disability benefits, call (800) 234-5772 and ask for Form SSA-7004-PC. A few weeks after returning the completed form, you will receive a Personal Earnings and Benefits Estimate Statement. Check it carefully for errors. Incorrect information could deprive you of rightful benefits.

Disability

Disability coverage usually starts with the fifth full month of disability and ends at age 65, when retirement benefits typically take over. You may have to file several appeals to get deserved benefits. A person must be on Social Security disability for 2 years before he or she will be covered by Medicare.

Representative payee

A Representative Payee is a person appointed by a Social Security recipient or the Social Security Administration (SSA) to manage a Social Security or Veterans' Administration benefit check if the recipient is unable to do so on their own behalf.

You can become a Representative Payee by completing a form at the SSA or VA office. Call the Social Security Administration at (800) 937-2000, or your local Social Security office.

Applying for benefits

Upon the death of a Social Security recipient, you must go to the local Social Security administration office to apply for benefits.

What to take when you apply

Take the decedent's:
• Original death certificate
• Original Social Security card
• W-2 form (if decedent was self-employed, take their last federal income tax return)
• Proof of divorce (if you are applying for benefits as a divorced spouse)

Benefit checks

Survivors are not allowed to keep the Social Security benefit check for the month in which the person died. If you keep these or subsequent checks, you will be responsible for reimbursement. (However, pension funds will typically allow you to retain the check in a similar situation.) You'll need to present to the SSA both the original death certificate and the original Social Security card to stop benefit checks for the deceased from arriving in the mail. The Social Security Act can change, so contact the nearest Social Security Administration for a full explanation of your current rights.

Where to request original documents

If you cannot find the original documents required to file a claim with the SSA, contact the city, county or state in which the birth or death took place. The Vital Statistics (also called Vital Records) department maintains records of births, deaths, marriages and divorce. (Get at least 2 copies of anything you order.)

Medicare

Started in 1965, Medicare is the Federal health insurance program for people 65 or older. Certain disabled people under 65 and people of any age who have permanent kidney failure are also eligible for Medicare coverage.

Medicare is divided into 2 parts:
• Part A (hospital insurance)
• Part B (medical insurance for doctors' charges in and out of the hospital)

You must make monthly payments, which are usually deducted from your Social Security check. In 1994, the deduction was $36.60.

Enrollment

To enroll in Medicare, contact the Social Security Administration 3 months before your 65th birthday. You have 6 months in which to sign up. (Look for the SSA phone number in your phone book under Social Security Administration or U.S. Government.)

Over 65 and still working

If you continue to work past the age of 65, and are part of an employer health plan, you should apply for Part A only. When you are no longer part of the employer health plan, you will have 6 months in which to purchase a supplemental insurance policy. At this point, a 6-month waiting period can be imposed if there is a pre-existing condition.

To learn the latest changes on coverage and cost, contact the American Association of Retired Persons, (202) 434-2277, or the Social Security Administration, (800) 772-1213.

Insurance recommendations:

• Don't pay for insurance in cash
• Don't over-insure yourself.
• Don't duplicate coverage. Even with additional insurance, you still may pay the deductible and co-payments.
• Do take advantage of the 10-15 day 'free look' period.
• Do review 'accident benefits only' insurance plans very carefully. Illnesses will not be covered.

Medicaid

Medicaid is a state and Federal program designed to provide financial relief to people with minimal assets and high medical costs. (The program is known by various names: in California, Medi-Cal; in Arizona, ALTCS). Because nursing home care is so expensive (currently about $40,000 per year in some states), even people of average means look to Medicaid for help.

Medicaid and Medicare are separate programs. Don't count on Medicare to pay for long-term care. It rarely pays for more than 20-100 days of care in a nursing home.

Financial eligibility

In most states, a single person is only allowed to have only $2,000 per year; you have to 'spend down' the rest to be eligible for Medicaid to pay your medical bills. Married people may keep much more, sometimes over $70,000. In addition, most Medicaid recipients are allowed to keep their home, furniture, one car and a savings account for funeral expenses.

Medicaid can penalize applicants who give away property in order to qualify for benefits. The government frowns on such maneuvers; applicants are checked to see if they have met the low-asset rule through a "look back" period. It is not true that you can give away $10,000 a year and still qualify. The $10,000 rule is for estate tax; it has nothing to do with Medicaid.

If you think the situation requires Medicaid, don't panic. Other don'ts: Don't give away houses or money. Don't falsify the Medicaid application. Instead, seek advice from a reliable source first before taking any important steps.

Good legal advice is crucial, since each state establishes different rules for Medicaid. The county Senior Legal Services and Local Legal Aid offices may be able to provide information or references for attorneys that specialize in Medicaid planning. For a list of elder law attorneys in your area, call (602) 881-4005.

To request the above list and the free booklet, *Questions and Answers When Looking for an Elder Law Attorney*, send a stamped, self-addressed envelope to:
National Academy of Elder Law Attorneys
655 N. Alvernon Way
Tucson, Arizona 85711

Questions to ask potential advisors:

- Have you ever seen a Medicaid application form for the state of (your state)?
- Have you ever appealed a Medicaid notice at a Fair Hearing?
- Have you ever advised a family with $_____ (provide the amount of money you have in savings or investments) in assets to plan for Medicaid? Did they qualify?
- How do you keep current on Medicaid changes?

If the advisor doesn't have good answers for these questions, reconsider using their services.

Steps to take

There are constant changes in Federal and state Medicaid laws. Depending upon the circumstances, families can benefit from planning for Medicaid by using the appropriate techniques:
- planned and documented 'spend down' of assets
- carefully timed gifts
- court orders
- special types of annuities
- irrevocable trusts
- special types of trusts (in rare situations)
- family limited partnerships

Important

The do-it-yourself approach to these techniques will usually backfire. Each approach works only when it is part of an overall plan, and should be used only after all the advantages and disadvantages have been considered.

Annuities

Don't be taken in by annuity salespeople who pressure seniors to buy annuities in order to qualify for Medicaid, and don't trust hucksters who want to sell 'Medicaid Qualifying Trusts' door-to-door. Seek a qualified advisor and ask them why a particular plan might work for you. Also, have the advisor explain the disadvantages of the plans.

Ask yourself if you really need or want Medicaid. You might consider other available sources such as long-term insurance,

Medicare coverage or the repositioning of assets. Another consideration: Do your doctors accept Medicaid?

Establish a Medicaid trust   The idea behind this restructuring of financial holdings is to give away your money so that you can keep it! You may also want to remind people, such as your parents, that they've worked hard and paid taxes for years, and now it's their turn to receive some help. Our health care system benefits those people who have or can create a low income, especially those faced with long-term care.

Plan carefully   A trust transfers property to another person to manage. The trick is to plan ahead (by at least 2 1/2 years before you apply for Medicaid). Otherwise, you may cause a 30-month waiting period to be used against you before either you or your spouse can qualify for Medicaid benefits. Another recent ruling allows your house to be seized if you don't transfer it properly.

Important   When contacting Medicaid, don't give your name or the patient's name. An inquiry may immediately start an account and establish an eligibility date.

In some circumstances, transferring assets makes sense, regardless of the penalty. This is because the length of ineligible penalty time is based on the amount of money you transferred divided by the average cost of nursing home care in your area. Hey, ask a lawyer about it.

The fees for setting up a Medicaid trust are between $1,000-3,000. Since the law varies in each state, it is essential to use an attorney who is familiar with your state's Medicaid law.

TIP: Read *The Medicaid Planning Handbook* by Alexander A. Bove, Jr.

Chapter 3

The Emotional Aspects

Remember You are perfect prey for emotional extortion. By having every-thing in order, you can keep the vultures at bay.

There are a wealth of books written about the emotional aspect of terminal illness and death. (A list of titles are located in Chapter 12). The following briefly touches upon some basic areas.

Note: To make this chapter easier to read, the term 'the person you love' is used for all forms of personal relationships: spouse, com-panion, child, sibling, relative or friend.

Four stages When the person you love becomes seriously ill or dies, you can expect to go through several stages of adjustment.

Stage 1: Shock and denial Shock and denial are common reactions to a painful reality.

In the case of a serious illness
If you are in denial, you are likely to rationalize away symptoms of severe illness. This defensive posture is a normal part of the adjustment process and is transitory; it cushions the blow of a harsh reality.

In the case of a death
You may find it may be impossible to believe that the person you love has really died.

Stage 2: Disorientation No longer unable to deny reality, you may become irrational. You are likely to feel anger and resentment. Empathetic support and assistance from other people will help you during this time.

In the case of a death
You are likely to feel abandoned and to hope that the person you love will return.

Stage 3: Anxiety and emotional expression As you begin to accept reality, you are likely to release powerful emotions, most likely anger and guilt.

In the case of a serious illness

The medical community is an alien environment where you are expected to communicate with people in a language you don't understand. Decisions abound.

In the case of a death

You may feel scared by the death of someone you love. Guilt from second-guessing and self-blame can be the most difficult aspects of grief to overcome. You may find it helpful to share your feelings with someone who understands, or to talk at length about the loss to a professional.

Stage 4: Adjustment

Time and information will help you through the acceptance process of a long-term illness or death.

In the case of a serious illness

Seek support and knowledge. Ask the physician how much the patient knows about their condition. Familiarize yourself with the medical world by calling on social workers, psychologists or clergy available at the hospital. Helpful resources include community crisis centers or private therapists.

In the case of a death

Grieving is the way we heal ourselves when someone we love has died. A feeling of diminished strength is part of the grieving process. You must let yourself grieve to preserve your health and be able to go on with life. You may need to cry for hours on end. Plan for more resting time; it takes a lot of energy to grieve.

Long-term illnesses and caregiving decisions

Seek help

You may need help from a financial adviser who has dealt with cases involving long-term illnesses. If your own attorney, accountant or insurance agent seem unfamiliar with the details, call an association for people with specific diseases, such as the local chapters of: the American Cancer Society, the Alzheimer's Disease Association, or AIDS organizations. Someone there may be able to refer you to an expert. (The phone numbers for many such organizations are listed in Chapter 11.)

Care Givers You alone cannot meet all the needs of a patient or an aging parent. The key to balancing your role and responsibilities as an effective care giver is a network of friends, family neighbors, volunteers, professional and paid helpers. For instance, a neighbor may be a welcome source of support and companionship.

The first step To start building your network, call the information clearinghouse for the specific disease or disability involved in your situation. (The phone numbers are listed in Chapter 11.)

Don't stress out—find help One of the prime causes of burnout is running errands. Take advantage of available services:

- Learn if a local pharmacy delivers free of charge.
- Free or low-cost rides are available to ailing or disabled individuals from a local seniors center or social services agency.
- Local universities with programs in social services may have students interested in an internship which may help you.

Several agencies can help you Examples: A home-health agency can help with shopping and cleaning; Meals-On-Wheels can provide a special food program.

Other resources:
- Local Area Agency for the Aging
- County health department
- Department of social services
- Jewish Family Services
- Catholic Social Services or other denominational support organizations

Support groups People with similar problems share their emotions and experiences, and together arrive at ways to be more successful with their ailing family members or friends. Local support groups can provide a crash course about long-term care.

You'll learn the basics, such as:
- Making ice chips available to the patient.
- Not pushing the patient to eat food.
- Expecting uncharacteristic behavior as a terminally ill person vents anger about their situation.

Responsibilities

Determine your areas of responsibility. This will help with the struggle to meet the needs of the patient, your family and yourself. You will no longer feel helpless as you gain a sense of control over your life. The feeling of being out of control creates stress. Whether or not the person you love acknowledges your presence, you are doing everything you can to brighten their days and make them feel that they are part of the living world. When they are gone, you will be glad you did everything you could. You can never relive those days.

Helpful hints to care givers

- Unrelenting optimism from others makes patients feel isolated.
- Acknowledge and discuss your feelings.
- Patients long for a chance to air their true feelings.
- Don't be overprotective.
- A velvet-glove treatment that avoids the 'bad news' of daily life leaves patients feeling unwanted and unneeded.
- Be informed and realistic about the patient's condition.
- Find a support group for the patient and for you.
- Take care of yourself. You can be of no help to the patient if you get ill.
- Keep family routines.
- Ask for help.
- Look to the future.

Long-distance care giving

The National Association of Private Geriatric Care Managers, (602) 881-8008, can make care giving from a long distance easier. You also may wish to contact your county's local area agency on aging for available services listed under "Geriatric Care" or "Older Adults Care Managers". Next time you visit, get a phone book for the city in which your ailing parent or the person you love lives.

Care managers

Care managers are usually part of private organizations; they provide services by social workers, nurses, etc. An initial visit— which may be all you need— ranges from $150-$350. Monthly fees can run as high as $400-500.

For a list of care managers in your state, and the state of your ill parent, send $3.00 to:
Children of Aging Parents (CAPS)
Woodbourne Office Campus
Suite 302-A
1609 Woodbourne Road
Levittown, PA 19057

Respite— the interval of rest or relief

There are various daycare centers for adults and children that provide respites for care givers. Public and private health agencies and in-home nursing services provide respite care for you and the person you are helping.

The Brookdale Center for Aging, at Hunter College in New York, (800) 648-2673, is a national clearing house for information regarding respite resources. Other sources for referrals include:
• city, county or state health departments
• childrens' social services
• local nursing registry
• hospital social services

Difficult decisions

If you are suddenly required to make decisions for someone whose illness has rendered them incompetent, the task may be overwhelming. If the person is comatose or terminally ill, a hospital's ethics committee can help with the issue of dying with grace and dignity.

Patients in a persistent vegetative state have permanent loss of consciousness. They are unaware of their surroundings and can no longer experience pain or pleasure. Some researchers have found that most Americans support a patient's right to die with dignity. Many people also fear and oppose the intrusion of life-support technology into one of life's most private moments. The difficult subject of how to make life and death decisions for someone you love is discussed further in Chapter 9.

Coping with a death

Death is an inescapable fact of life. Because of the psychological issues typically left unresolved, some of the basic problems include guilt and remorse.

Seek help for yourself when coping with a death:
- Seek support from community bereavement groups.
- Consider psychotherapy; protracted grief responds well to treatment.
- Look into anti-depressants; great strides have been made in the past 5 years.

People who make an effort to resolve issues before the death of someone they love are often rewarded. These issues include learning about family history, confronting unresolved problems, understanding a person's importance in your life, and gaining more sympathy and understanding of parents as people. You won't change history, but you can get rid of a lot of frustration.

Never saying "I love you" to a parent is high up on the list of regrets people have once a parent dies. Whatever you would like to tell someone on their deathbed, say to them today. You may never get another chance.

Important

Twelve ways to ease emotional pain and depression:
1. Get dressed every day.
2. Get out of the house at least once a day, regardless of what

you do once you step into the fresh air.

3. Bring green plants, flowers or pets into your home. Living things force you to think of life.
4. Stay in the sunlight as much as possible, especially in winter.
5. Exercise every day. Exercise acts as a buffer against stress and can help protect the cardiovascular and immune systems from the effects of stressful events. Taking control of your health also offers psychological benefits. (Many bereaved people claim exercise is the most helpful thing they do.)
6. Plan activities that oblige you to attend. Volunteer your time.
7. Structure your day so you don't have an excess of time with nothing to do.
8. Don't do any one thing for more than an hour.
9. Clean out your closets and drawers to avoid turning them a 'shrine' for your spouse or child.
10. Spend time with children. They'll force your thoughts into the sunshine.
11. Don't allow self-pity. The moment this emotion occurs, do something kind for someone less fortunate.
12. Be gentle with yourself— see a movie, have a massage, shop, attend a sporting event. Don't set your expectations too high.

Feeling alone

The primary source of human anxiety is feeling alone. The most powerful emotions are efforts to avoid the psychological 'prison' of being alone.

There are four seasons of grieving

The 'firsts' will be the most difficult: the first Thanksgiving, the first anniversary. Each season brings up memories that can temporarily intensify the sense of loss. Expect grief to come in waves that subside as time passes. Adaptation is eventually achieved as grief fades into warm memories.

Coping with the 'empty chair' during the holiday season

Planning is the key to successfully coping with the holidays. A change in pattern can be good.

Mental preparation for social events	• Balance solitude with social times. Solitude can renew strength.
	• Schedule time to grieve. When you have set aside some time for grieving, you'll find it easier to control your flow of grief in public.
	• Before attending a social event, remember to plan what you'll wear, who you'll see and how you'll return home. Plan ahead — not at a moment of weakness— and you'll do a better job of it.
	• Confront the conspiracy of silence. People may not mention your spouse or child's name for fear of upsetting you. Tell your family and friends that it is important for you to talk about the person you love during the holiday season; this is when your spouse, child or friend is very much on your mind.
	• Minimize the use of alcohol. Excessive consumption of alcohol will only increase depression.
	• People want to know what is helping you to cope and what isn't. Be truthful.
	• Understand that you will experience a nearly universal anxiety that the choice you made was the wrong one.
	• Relive happy memories. Pick three special memories of past times with your loved one. Recall them often, especially if outbursts of grief occur at inappropriate times.
Holiday traditions	• Change traditions. Hold holiday gatherings at a different place this year.
	• Don't be pressured by anyone to participate in the holidays.
	• Don't send holiday cards if you would rather not. It's a lot of work.
	• Don't bother putting up a Christmas tree by yourself this year. It won't be wonderful.
	• If decorating or buying gifts is too difficult for you to do this year, ask a friend to do it for you. Or don't decorate or shop at all; it's your decision to make.
Family	• Don't forget the rest of the family. Listen to them. Talk to them, especially the children.
	• If you want to be alone, just tell the appropriate people that you

won't be joining them this year. Or tell one person and have them relay information to the others.

New holiday activities

- Go to a movie.
- Write notes to people who have been especially nice.
- Rent a video.
- Watch or attend a sporting event.
- Take someone special shopping.
- Find a new creative outlet.
- Contribute to, or work with, a group that your spouse or friend supported. Use the money that you would have spent on a gift for your spouse, friend or child to buy a gift for someone he or she cared about.
- Adopt a needy family or volunteer at a community center. People that you don't know need you.
- Work your way through a list of 20 favorite activities.
- Seek the company of enjoyable people.

Emotional release

Laughter and crying (for females; males would prefer to be thrown off a building...) are the most effective natural releases of the painful emotions of fear, anger and sadness. Ranting and raving help to release the tensions of frustration and anger, too. You may find relief by screaming in your car while driving alone; to the outside world you'll appear to be singing. Punching a heavy bag or pillow, or spending an hour in a batting cage is also very useful. Rent a movie that makes you cry. Be aware of how much energy is released during crying, and how tired— but clear— you'll feel when you've finished.

People who hold in their frustration and anger usually develop guilt. Depression can often occur if you fail to acknowledge or discuss your sadness; but depression (if not too severe) can also deepen your personality, leaving you better able to cope with future problems. Grief is often combined with anger and fear. It is healthiest to express your feelings— and forgive yourself—

because anger and guilt that you do not release can turn into hostility and resentment.

It takes time to accept a loss. Losing a spouse usually translates into 200-300 hours of tears. Such a 'healing timetable' can take one to two years or more. Feeling unexpectedly angry or scared is often a sign that you have not consciously recognized a loss. It helps to remember that pain is inevitable when you love people.

Chapter 4

Failing Health and Lifestyle Changes

Loss of independence

Driving represents independence for many people. If you think your parent should no longer drive, enroll the help of a doctor to express his or her medical opinion. Chances are the unpleasant truth will be more palatable coming from a third party.

To deflect the loss of independence, suggest different modes of transportation: group cab or limo rides, train trips, buses, county 'ride' programs, or rides from friends or relatives.

'Quality of Life'

To determine what a person really wants in terms of 'quality of life', you must talk to them about resuscitation, tube feeding and wills. It's also important to discuss these issues with health care providers. You can avoid many problems if you choose an attending physician based on, in part, the doctor's feelings about resuscitation, life support, artificial nutrition and hydration. These issues are also important when selecting a nursing home.

One of the caregiver's important responsibilities is to suggest that a will be updated, or made if none exists. Chapter 1 discusses other legal matters that should be addressed.

Last requests

Discussions about funerals are generally considered in poor taste at best; however, very old or very sick people may find comfort in planning a funeral that carries out their wishes. The discussion may actually be much less painful than you expect. Ask if a burial plot has been purchased and, if so, where the deed to the plot is kept. Ask if a specific religious funeral service or secular (non-religious) memorial service is desired. If no plans exist, you may do some research into local funeral facilities so you don't have to decide at a more difficult time. (For more details, see Chapter 10.)

Chapter 5

Medical Facilities, the Medical Community, Hospital Care and Visiting a Patient

Hospitals

In selecting a hospital, determine which facility in your area provides the best care for a specific condition. If you live near a city, you should consider a university-affiliated 'teaching hospital' with sophisticated equipment and an extensive staff of medical specialists. You also may wish to consider a 'sentinel' hospital such as the Mayo Clinic in Rochester, Minnesota, or Memorial Sloan-Kettering Cancer Center in New York City; they can provide excellent medical care or refer you to a first-rate doctor or hospital in your area.

The other side of the coin

When selecting a facility, remember that people who are sick are sometimes reluctant to travel long distances from their home and family, especially if traffic conditions are difficult. Family members may find it difficult to make patient visits. And, realistically, not all major cities have 'teaching hospitals'. The downside of a 'teaching hospital' is the amount of poking, probing and staring that the patient must endure. Many older people, especially when quite ill, resent having ten or fifteen different physicians examining them. Therefore, most patients end up at the hospital where their personal physicians practice.

Check-in

Patients should take:
- toothbrush and toothpaste
- comb or brush
- razor and shaving equipment
- front-opening coat-style robe (mark or sew in a label in case it gets 'misplaced')
- comfortable slippers

- reading glasses and reading material (leave contact lenses at home; attach a small name tag to your glasses)

plus:

- health insurance identification card
- insurance forms
- Medicare and/or Medicaid cards (if applicable)

Leave personal possessions and money behind, especially jewelry; theft happens in hospitals. To ensure compliance with the patient's wishes, fill out and take a Durable Power of Attorney for Health Care and a Living Will form. You must advise the doctor of the patient's wishes about life support, etc., before the patient's condition makes discussion impossible.

Important

Make sure a close family member has the phone number of the patient's attending physician. Many times the patient is too sick or uncomfortable to ask the proper questions or demand proper care during the doctor's brief visits. Pain medication and other drugs often interfere with the patient's ability to think clearly. Communicating with the patient's physician also lets the doctor know that you expect the best of care.

Anesthesiology

Before surgery, make your anesthesiologist aware of any:
- capped teeth
- stomach upset brought about by anesthesia in the past
- existing medical conditions that require antibiotics or other special care

Special services

Many hospitals offer special services to acquaint you with their facility. These services may include the Human Support Department, Chaplain's Office, Crisis Intervention Service, Discharge Planners, and Patient Hotlines.

You can also order a 24-hour private nurse to care for a patient, at your own cost.

Visiting a patient	Give the patient the pleasure of anticipating your visit; let him or her know when you'll visit.

TIP: Most patients prefer receiving mail to all else.

What to take with you

Favored gift items include:
- note paper and/or stamps
- books with large print
- hand-size photo album with family photos

Conversation

The sterile appearance of medical facilities is enough to stifle anyone. If this is your reaction, explain to the patient that it is a little difficult to act yourself in these surroundings. Mention that you would like to be able to enjoy the time together as you typically have in the past.

Questions

These are helpful questions you can ask:
- What kinds of visitors, entertainment or conversations would you like to have?
- What do you miss?
- What do you need from me? (Tell them you feel insecure in your role as a caregiver.)
- Is there is anything I can help someone at home with? (This questions is sure to bring pleasure and relief to a patient with a spouse at home.)
- Would you like me to update you on my life? (This provides the patient with a distraction from their situation and gives them a sense of purpose.)
- Do you have any advice?
- How does it feel when the discomfort starts and when the pain subsides?
- What physical changes and challenges do you have?
- On a scale of 1 to 10, with 10 being terrific, how do you feel emotionally today? Ask the same question again, but

substitute the word 'physically' for 'emotionally.' (If you're really organized, you may want to keep a little chart.)
- How often does your doctor visit you?
- What is your doctor telling you about your prognosis and the treatment you'll receive?
- Do you agree with your doctor?

Recommendations
- Discuss the hopes and fears they're experiencing.
- To get your parent to talk openly about what's happening, you can try to get the conversation going by saying: "You look tired, Mom." or "You're getting weaker, aren't you, Dad?"
- Listening is much more supportive than changing the subject or giving pep talks.
- At times, "I'm here" may be the two most supportive words you can say.

You might learn from children who, when asked, said they would treat someone who has been sick for a long time by:
- Staying by their side.
- Treating them like they're rich

TIP: If there is a choice about physical therapy, choose to start as soon as possible.

Patient rights

Understand that when someone you love becomes a defenseless patient, you become the defender of that patient's rights. The Patients' Bill of Rights is recognized by the American Hospital Association. If a patient advocate is available at the hospital, you can seek his or her advice. A patient advocate functions as an official liaison between the medical community and the rest of the world. For instance, after the third unsuccessful try at finding a patient's vein with a needle, a nurse is required to ask for help from another nurse. A patient has the right to refuse any recommended medical treatment and the right to request a second medical opinion. (Be aware that some insurance companies will not pay for second opinions; however, some will pay with pre-authorization.) The nursing manager of the unit may be able to answer your questions.

Patient discharge

After discharge, if further care is needed at home, the hospital's case manager or social services department can arrange for:

• services at home
• a transfer to another health care facility
• specialty services
• other options for continued care

Don't be shocked if these services aren't covered by your insurance policy. Many insurance companies pay only minimal post-hospital expenses. Insist that your physician work with you to get as many services paid for as possible. Note that primary physicians are more cooperative on this point than surgeons, for example.

A medical social worker can help with:
• the acceptance and adjustment to a disability
• chronic conditions
• referrals to community resources

Some hospitals offer special discussion/support group programs through their social services and utilization management departments to help people cope with specific, chronic illnesses. Others have specific programs for pain management, psychological and rehabilitation therapy, and other non-medical techniques such as physician-administered acupuncture.

Premature discharge   Upon admission as a Medicare patient, the patient should receive a sheet titled "An Important Message from Medicare", which states, "According to Federal law, your discharge date must be determined solely by your medical needs and not by 'DRGs' (diagnostic related groups) or Medicare payments." Medicare patients are entitled to a written "discharge plan" and discharge planning services. It's illegal for hospitals to tell a patient to leave without determining if there is a safe home environment that is suitable for the patient's current condition. Recuperative alternatives include swingbeds (found in smaller hospitals) for custodial-level care or ANDs (administratively necessary days) that Medicare may pay for when a patient should be in a nursing home, but no bed is available. In both cases, the attending physician must certify the need for care; otherwise, Medicare won't pay.

If you think the patient is being prematurely discharged, you can:
• talk with your physician
• ask to see the hospital's patients' representative
• protest to the Peer Review Organization (PROs), a monitoring organization of doctors set up by federal law. (They are not located in the hospital.)

Medicare has a formal procedure to complain to the PRO. If you cannot reach your state's PRO, call Office of Medical Review, Health Standards and Quality Bureau, (301) 966-6851.

Several Medicare advocacy agencies can provide helpful information in the case of premature discharge:
• Legal Assistance to Medicare Patients — (203) 423-2556
• Legal Counsel for the Elderly — (202) 833-6720
• National Senior Citizens Law Center — (202) 887-5280
• Center for Medicare Advocacy — (203) 456-7790

TIP:	Send for *"Knowing Your Rights"* (Stock #D12330), AARP, 1909 K Street, NW, Washington, DC 20049. (Written specifically for Medicare carriers, but helpful for everyone.)

Payment

Carefully go over your hospital bill; hospitals are notorious for making errors and overcharging. Don't accept a charge such as: Pharmacy $642.00. Ask for an itemization.

For patients with Medicare, remember the billing order: Medicare is billed first, then any secondary carriers (such as group coverage), and then the patient, for the balance and any deductibles or co-payments.

Some hospitals have financial counselors who can answer questions concerning your medical and hospital insurance coverage. You have the right to appeal adverse decisions concerning Medicare coverage and reimbursement. Some hospitals will write off a percentage of your bill if you are unable to pay.

Hospital ethics committees

Most hospitals have ethics committees that can provide guidance, should you wish it, when you are faced with a life and death issue. They can help you decide what is in the patient's best interest.

'Code Blue'

Do-not-resuscitate (DNR). This is an order that can be filed in a patient's medical record to withhold cardiopulmonary resuscitation. Also called "no code". Discuss this issue with the attending physician. Obviously, a "no code" should be discussed at length with the patient; it is their decision to make. Ensure that the necessary forms are completed and that everyone is notified about the decision.

Chapter 6

Doctors

A doctor can be the best resource for helping you build a 'support system' of professionals and agencies.

How to find them	Although you may think friends or co-workers are the best source of medical referrals, the most sensible way to find a new doctor is to consider one's medical needs first. Determine what area of expertise would be of greatest benefit. If you or the person you are helping is healthy, you might pick a doctor who is board-certified in one of the four key specialties: family practice, pediatrics, gynecology or internal medicine.
Sources	You may wish to contact an appropriate hospital in your area or county medical society to request the names of several board-certified doctors who might consider accepting a new patient. Nurses are a good unofficial source of information.
Older patients	If the patient is elderly, be careful to find a physician that the patient can trust. If a patient does not have confidence and trust in their physician, they may have difficulty recovering from an illness or surgery. A hospital can provide you with referrals; ask for: geriatric services, human resources or discharge counseling. Churches and synagogues often have referral lists. The National Association of Professional Geriatric Care Managers can tell you how to contact its members in your area; call (602) 881-8008.
Physicians in good standing	To learn if a doctor has ever been officially sanctioned for misconduct, contact the Public Citizen Health Research Group, 200 P St. NW, Washington, DC 20036. To verify a doctor's board certification, call the American Board of Medical Specialties at (800) 776-2378.

What to look for	Contact each doctor on your 'consideration' list and set up a brief interview, either by phone or in person. (Be aware that you may be asked to pay for an appointment.) Some of the best specialists are very busy and an interview may be impossible to arrange.
Questions to ask the doctor:	• What approach would you take if a patient developed an incurable ailment? A doctor who is willing to help patients explore alternative treatments is best. • What would you do if a patient had a medical crisis such as a heart attack? You want someone who can get the best cardiologist, cardiac surgeons and a bed in a first-rate cardiac intensive care unit. • Would you honor a patient's request for (a) no artificial life support, (b) full life support?
	The best-suited doctor is generally the professional who has the most experience in treating a disorder that a patient has or will likely develop. Bias your selection toward the optimistic doctor and one who is willing to solicit information from other doctors or specialists. These 'mini-consults' with other doctors can often be accomplished by phone and will reduce your expenses.
HMOs and PPOs	The options are somewhat limited in the case of insurance plans with member doctors and hospitals. Select a health maintenance organization (HMO), preferred provider organization (PPO), or other managed health-care plan based on the reputation of the available doctors and hospitals. When selecting an individual member physician, use the same principles as stated previously.
How to communicate	Arrange a meeting with the attending physician to learn about a patient's medical condition; you may have to be persistent, especially if the patient is in a hospital.

A patient may want 'another set of ears' in the room to remember and interpret detailed or unwelcome information. (This strategy applies to hospital and office visits.)

Take notes and/or a tape recorder to remember what was discussed. People tend to get nervous and forgetful in the presence of a 'white coat'. Don't be intimidated by doctors and nurses; even when you're in the hospital, it's still your body.

When consulting a doctor, bring a list of:
• questions
• symptoms
• goals

Between visits with your doctor, jot down questions you would like answered.

Questions to ask include:
• Can you predict how successful the operation or treatments will be?
• What are the risks of this treatment?
• Will there be much pain?
• How will it be controlled?
• How often does the doctor do this type of surgery?
• How often does the hospital host this type of surgery?
• Who can I talk to about a special concern I have?
• What resources in the community are available to me?
• How can I learn more about my condition?
• What should I tell my relatives and friends?
• What long-term side effects can I expect?
• How will long-term side effects affect my daily activities? And quality of life?

Request copies of test results, consultations and other elements of your medical record. It may help to read and evaluate findings at home. Don't be rushed or pressured into making major health decisions.

Second opinions	Don't worry about hurting your doctor's feelings by getting a second or third opinion. Insist on taking previous test results with you to the second-opinion doctor to avoid delays, 'lost' results, and/or going through a battery of tests again.

Complaints

If a patient has a complaint about a doctor regarding lack of information or treatment, etc., the following professionals or groups may help:

- a hospital's patient representative
- a hospital social worker
- bioethics consultants
- a hospital's ombudsmen
- a hospital's ethics committee
- the hospital administrator
- social workers
- insurance companies
- attorneys

You must initiate claims of medical malpractice within a given period of time (each state varies). Your local bar association can give you the names of attorneys who can explain your state law. Check your phone listings for the Medical Board Physician Complaint Unit.

Payment

TIPS: Always keep a copy of anything mailed to a doctor, hospital or insurance company.

Ask if discounts are given for cash payments.

Physicians

Doctors sometimes underestimate what insurance will cover. If your insurance will not cover a great portion of a bill, ask your doctor if he or she will accept the insurance or Medicare payment as payment in full. You may be surprised at their response. For backup, you may call other doctors to learn what they charge for comparable services.

Labs   Some lab facilities will agree to accept insurance payments (i.e. 80% coverage) as payment in full if the request is made in advance. If necessary, suggest that you are considering the use of other diagnostic facilities. Example: the cost for MRIs vary considerably between labs.

Hospitals   For hospitalization, Medicare and HMO/PPO patients need to check with their surgeon or admitting doctor to make sure that other providers of services (radiologists, anesthesiologists, pathologists, pain care management, etc.) are members of your insurance group or a Medicare participating physician. This step can greatly reduce out of pocket expenses.

PPOs (Preferred Provider Organizations)   When you receive your bill, always make sure the proper adjustments (write-offs) have been made.

Medicare-participating vs non-participating providers   Non-participating providers (also known as non-accept assignment physicians) will bill Medicare. Medicare will pay the physician a set limit. The patient is responsible for the balance.

Participating providers (also known as accept assignment physicians) will bill Medicare and accept Medicare's payment as 'payment in full', as long as the deductible has been met. Participating physicans have agreed to write off any balance and not bill the patient any remaining costs.

TIP: A doctor may accept an assignment if asked, even if he or she is non-participating.

If you don't have insurance   Remind your doctor that medical care is a financial burden for you and your family. Many doctors will give courtesy discounts. Family doctors and internists will sometimes ask specialists to reduce their fees as a favor to the referring doctor. You may be able to qualify for the Hill-Burton Uncompensated Services program through your hospital.

Payment schedules   Always call and set up a payment schedule if you have financial difficulties; don't ignore medical bills. A payment of only $10 per month will show your intent to pay and will probably forestall any collection agency attempts, especially if the payment schedule is pre-arranged.

TIP: When making payment arrangements, remember to note the date and name of the person that made the agreement with you.

Opportunities   To get the most from your insurance coverage and make sure items are 'payable', ask your doctors to write a prescription for everything they recommend. Send a copy of the prescription and receipt to your insurance carrier.

If your insurance company rejects a claim, your doctor can write a letter to your insurer explaining:
• why your case is unusual and requires extra care.
• why it is cost-effective to get the extra treatment or services now, rather than later.
• the details of your condition, treatment plan and duration on treatment.

Chapter 7

Long-Term Care

Only 5 percent of people sixty-five and older live in a nursing home.

The other 95% employ a wide range of living arrangements, including:
- adult day care
- adult foster homes
- board and care or adult homes
- congregate housing, co-housing
- continuing care retirement communities (CCRCs)
- elder cottage housing opportunity (ECHO) homes
- enriched housing
- group homes
- home care
- hospice care
- housing for the elderly
- public housing for senior citizen
- respite care
- retirement communities
- senior centers shared housing

Nursing home care

If a nursing home is the best choice, three levels of nursing home care are available:

- skilled nursing facilities (SNF)
- intermediate care facilities (ICF)
- custodial or residential care facilities (RCF)

Because skilled nursing care is provided by licensed nurses, SNFs are the most expensive choice. Skilled care is the only level of care for which Medicare will reimburse, and then only a limited amount of coverage is provided. You may wish to consider purchasing the lowest level of care necessary.

Which facility?	For resources and referrals, contact local social workers, senior centers (listed in the county or city section of the phone book), the Department of Social Services, or religious affiliations, and ask them to recommend case managers or brokers. The rules for Medicare and Medicaid reimbursement are complex. The administrators of the facilities you are considering can help you determine a person's financial resources.
Ask the professionals	You should ask the attending physician for recommendations. Take into consideration that a doctor may limit his or her visits to various nursing homes. You may have to change doctors if your patients's physician doesn't visit the facility that you have selected.
	Many books explain the details of nursing home care and selection. Several recommended books are listed in Chapter 12.
Informative brochures	To help you select a nursing or retirement facility, you can get brochures from:

California Association of Health Facilities
1401 21st St., Suite 202
Sacramento, CA 95814
(916) 444-7600

AARP Fulfillment
P.O. Box 22796
Long Beach, CA 90801-5796
Request D13803 — *Care Management: Arranging for Long Term Care*

What to expect	Nursing-home residents have rights (which vary with each state):

• the right to choose a personal physician
• the right to choose a roommate
• the right to consult one's own medical records.

For more information, contact:

National Citizen's Coalition for Nursing Home Reform
1224 M St., NW
Washington, DC 20005
(202) 393-2018

National Senior Citizen's Law Center
1815 H Street, NW
Washington, DC 20006
(202) 887-5280

Important

At any facility, you would be surprised how much time is spent by family and friends performing caregiving chores, relative to the time health-care professionals spend.

When considering a facility, ask to see their written policy on psychotropic drugs and restraints. In general, the policy should state that psychotropic drugs cannot be administered to a resident without the written consent of either the resident or certain designated family members. Restraints should be permitted only when the resident is in danger of harming themselves or others.

Visiting

As people get older, they need occasions to anticipate. Visit regularly and schedule your visits. It takes about 6 months for an aged person to acclimate to new accommodations. Your presence can reduce the patient's loneliness, and your visits let the staff know that you're watching how residents are being treated. Introduce yourself to the staff and talk to them on every visit. And when you leave, be sure to let your loved one know when you're coming again.

Keys to good visits

- Plan your conversations. Mention a planned event that your parent can look forward to.
- Spend at least half an hour visiting. Arrive on time and tell your parent how long you can stay.

- Older people may have difficulty seeing or hearing. Sit close or pull up a chair.
- When talking, give the other person a pat. People need physical contact.
- Go outside for a walk. Movement helps to refresh the body and mind.
- Bring a surprise. A plant, fresh fruit, a letter from a mutual friend, a magazine, a photo or a book can be the focus of conversation.
- Ask about the past. Older people enjoy reminiscing.
- Ask about unfinished business. Ask if there is anyone else they want to see and if there are any tasks they want you to perform.
- Bring a child or small pet. Children and pets add a dimension of happiness and hope.
- You can involve other residents in your visits if your parent likes the idea. This approach helps develop relationships that can be enjoyed when you're not there.
- Don't be afraid to say things such as "I love you" or "When you die, I'll miss you". It is easier to say these things now than to wish later that you had.

Gifts for long-term care seniors:	• Assorted greeting cards
	• Books with large print
	• Calendars
	• Cordless phone
	• Phone with touch tone, adjustable volume control, and/or phone number memory
	• Phone for hearing impaired
	• Crossword puzzle book and a crossword puzzle dictionary
	• Gourmet coffee or tea
	• Telephone company gift certificate
	• Restaurant gift certificates
	• Storage unit for under the bed
	• Cassette tape of favorite short story, novel or classic (if you read well, tape it yourself)

- Orthopedic pillow
- Photo album, hand-size, with family photos inside
- Cassettes of old radio shows
- Divided plastic pillbox
- Pill cutter
- T-shirt with a picture of grandchildren printed on the front

TIPS: Don't forget humor. See Chapter 13 for a free one-month video-cassette rental of old Candid Camera shows.

A special gift that can't be purchased: soak a person's hands in warm soapy water, then clean and file their fingernails. Nail polish optional. Wash their face, brush their hair and clean their eyeglasses. Soak their feet in sudsy water and give them a foot massage. Finally, gently stretch their legs and arms. All the while talking or quietly enjoying each other's company.

Request *"What Every Caregiver Ought to Know"*. Send a self-addressed stamped envelope to: Commerce Clearing House, 4025 West Peterson Ave., Chicago, Illinois 60646.

Chapter 8

Home Care

Levels of care

Home health agencies can help you evaluate the type of help that you'll need. Levels of independent living and custodial care include:

- living alone with outside help
- shared living with independence
- group homes and retirement living
- living with family
- nursing homes
- AIDS board and care facilities

Selecting an agency

Know your needs so you don't purchase more care than necessary. Ask the prospective home care agency about unexpected charges, such as higher rates during evenings and weekends. Available services range from cooking and cleaning to full nursing care at home.

To avoid problems, seek an accredited or licensed agency. Get referrals from the National League for Nursing or the Joint Commission on the Accreditation of Health Care Organizations. Hospices and geriatric case managers can also help find extra services for you. (Look in the phone directory for Medical Management Consultants.) Typically, a doctor must arrange for services such as therapy, part-time home nursing care and special meals, etc.

Read *The Home Care Health Care Solution: A Complete Consumer Guide* by Janet Zhun Nassif.

You may want to order AARP's home-care program for family care givers. Home Is Where the Care Is includes 5 audio cassettes and a binder workbook. It's available from MTPS/AV Sales Library, 5000 Park Street North, St. Petersburg, FL 33709.

Special programs

Meals on Wheels and other food service programs may delay a person's need for a nursing home for many years. They deliver one hot meal a day to a person's home. The price is nominal and often based on one's ability to pay.

Homemaker services include assistance with grooming and dressing, and help with meal preparation, food shopping and light housekeeping. The cost is usually $10 per hour. Contact your Area Agency on Aging for information. (See the Local Government section of your phone book.)

Ask the patient's doctor to write a prescription for everything that he or she recommends. Take the prescriptions to a medical supply store (one that offers free delivery) and set up an account. Or your doctor can make the initial contact for you. The following organizations offer a mail-order service that can provide the medicines you need at slightly lower prices than a pharmacy:

American Association of Retired Persons
(800) 456-2277

Family Pharmaceuticals
(800) 922-3444

Medi-Mail
(800) 331-1458

If the patient needs a hospital bed, consider renting an all-electric bed, even though Medicare will not reimburse the full amount. Also consider upgrading to a lightweight wheelchair. Most people consider the upgrades worth the price difference. Be aware that you can rent walkers, rather than purchasing them. Ask your hospital representative to contact you before they purchase equipment for the patient; you may prefer to rent it.

Additional services

Although home care agencies can offer assistance, the bulk of the responsibility is in the hands of the patient's family and friends. They are the ones who will perform most of the nursing, feeding, bathing and pain control tasks.

Don't wait too long to seek help

Most care givers have a tendency to wait too long before seeking outside help. Consequences include:

- creating a situation where a highly dependent individual accepts assistance from only one person
- realizing help is needed, but making a hasty decision in desperation
- becoming too tired to be as helpful, patient or loving as you would like to be
- denying yourself many meaningful things, such as large family gatherings or weekend getaways

Other resources

To avoid injury to you or your loved one, you must not pretend knowledge of caregiving tasks. Instead, contact the resources below to get more information.

- *Local senior citizen center or social service agency.* Ask if any one is giving a brief course on how to take care of a dependent person.
- *Favorite nurse or physical therapist.* Ask them to show you how to lift and turn a person properly.
- *Local hospital or fire station.* Ask if they give first-aid courses.

TIPS:	For more information, send for *What Every Caregiver Ought to Know*, along with a self-addressed stamped envelope to: Commerce Clearing House, 4025 West Peterson Ave., Chicago, Illinois 60646.

Also, send a postcard to request:
A Handbook About Care in the Home, (order # D955), available from AARP, 601 E Street, NW, Washington, D.C. 20049.

More services Look for local senior information and referral agencies in your telephone directory under 'Seniors'. Be sure the organization is a non-profit, no-fee agency authorized by your local government or the Area Agency on Aging.

Contact your local, county, or state welfare or human services agencies; the American Red Cross or United Way, for programs which include:

- *Adopt-a-grandparent programs*—Weekly volunteer visitors.
- *Dial-a-Ride*— A transportation program.
- *ECHO Housing*—Elder Cottage Housing Opportunity units are small, self-contained, portable housing units that can be placed in the back- or side-yard of a single family house. First manufactured in Australia to enable parents to remain near their adult children.
- *Friendly Visiting*— A program in which individuals regularly look in on a household.
- *Grandma and Grandpa Sitting Service*— Programs frequently found in college communities with students interested in volunteer or hourly-fee work, home repairs, running errands, etc.
- *Home adaptation*— Low-interest loans available for changes to your home to accommodate wheelchairs, etc.
- *Home chore services*— Household cleaning, household repairs, and yard work.

- *Home health care*—A wide variety of medical services provided by nurses, physical therapists, social workers, nutritionists, and health aides.
- *Homemaker services*— Assistance with meals or housework.
- *Home sharing*— A resident manager and a few older people share housing and expenses.
- *Nutrition services*—Provides people with inexpensive, nutritious meals in group settings. Transportation may be provided.
- *Postal alert programs*— Letter carriers phone a designated person if they see signs of trouble. Free through a Red Cross or United Way office.
- *Respite care*—Available through some community groups; provides needed breaks for care givers.
- *Shopping services*—Grocery and pharmaceutical items delivered to residences.
- *Special transportation services*— Vehicles equipped to handle wheelchairs and other devices for people with limited mobility.
- *Special health aids or devices*—Availability of walkers, geriatric chairs, artificial limbs, etc.
- *Telephone reassurance*— A system devised to eliminate the risk of total isolation for elderly people living alone.

Medicare Medicare offers home care benefits for *homebound elderly*. In fact, because of the growing need, 50% of all internists and family practitioners now make house calls. For referrals, call your state medical society or the American Academy of Home Care Physicians at (410) 730-1623. Medicare currently reimburses from $27.50 to $50 for each home visit.

Payable services Telephone lifeline programs provide financial assistance to low-income Americans of all ages to help pay for telephone service.

Give services as gifts Give services, such as window cleaning and spring cleaning, as gifts. These services are listed in the yellow pages of your phone book.

Chapter 9

Taking Care of Final Matters

Prior to the last 50 years of modern medical technology, people usually died in their homes, cared for by their families. Today, most people don't realize that they can take care of family members themselves and that very ill people don't have to die in a hospital. The hospice movement is evidence of the awareness that death is a natural part of the life cycle. Prolonging life is not always in the dying person's best interest.

The question of where to die can become complicated. For many people, the choices are as follows:

• Home care without outside help.
• Home care with nurses or help from other professionals.
• Hospital care.
• Care at a hospice center.
• Nursing home care.

Hospice

A hospice is a facility or organization that provides pain relief and other support services for terminally-ill people and their families. Hospice care may be covered to some extent by insurance coverage and/or Medicare. In other cases, the services are free and covered by donations.

Services include:
• doctor and nursing services
• counseling, medical supplies and appliances
• physical and speech therapy
• medical social services
• home health aid and homemaker services
• physical and speech therapy

- pain management
- respite care (temporary relief for the caregiver)
- bereavement counseling

Eligibility

Hospice care also can be provided in a patient's home. To be eligible, the following conditions must be met:
- The patient is certified terminally ill by a physician, with a life expectancy of about six months or less.
- The patient has chosen to receive hospice benefits instead of the standard Part A and Part B Medicare benefits.
- The agency providing hospice care is certified by Medicare.
- A primary caregiver is available (relative or friend) to assume responsibility for custodial care and to make decisions.

For more information about hospice programs, call (800) 658-8898, or write to the National Hospice Organization, 1901 North Moore St., Suite 901, Arlington, VA 22209. To locate a childrens' hospice, call Children's Hospice International at (800) 242-4453.

Choosing to die at home

If a family member chooses to die at home, a nurse or hospice representative will teach you and the other caregivers everything you'll need to know. They help people cope with the physical and emotional pain of dying from a clearly terminal illness. If you work with a hospice, they will tell you not to call 911 if you don't want heroic life-saving measures taken at the end. The hospice will give you their emergency phone number. If you're not using a hospice, ask the attending doctor for his or her emergency phone number.

Organ donations

People interested in donating their body for research or donating organs can order a free Uniform Donor Card from the following organizations:

Living Bank, P.O. Box 6725, Houston, TX 77265
(713) 528-2971 or (800) 528-2971

Medic Alert, P. O. Box 1009, Turlock, CA 95381-1009
(209) 668-3333 or (800) 432-5378

National Society for Medical Research, 1000 Vermont Avenue,
Washington, DC 20005

Pain   Most people are concerned about the pain of death. Fortunately, attitudes about pain control/maintenance have changed. Today, pain is much more controllable due to new ideas about drug management. In some cases, access to drugs is controlled by the patients themselves, alleviating anxiety about alerting a nurse.

Near the end   Hopefully, long before a person is near death, all their last wishes are known and their pertinent papers are in order.

To help a terminally ill person clear up unfinished business, ask:
• Is there is anything special I can do for you?
• Would you like to see specific people?
• Would you like to reminisce about the past?
• Would you like to speak with the clergy about a personal matter?

Give reassurance   For instance, when a terminally ill person asks, 'How will (your mother) get along without me?' Reassure your father that you'll take care of Mom for him.

Common thoughts that go through a terminally ill person's mind are:
• How shall I best live the remainder of my life?
• How shall I die?
• How shall I have people remember me?

Last words   When a person is close to death, and you aren't sure they can hear or understand you, your voice may give them great comfort. You can say, "You're tired of being here. You're ready to go, aren't you?" "I'll miss you." "I love you."

Most people who have had the courage to help someone make the transition out of life find it a gratifying experience and consider their involvement a privilege.

Don't avoid the grieving process The death of a person you love or were caring for will release you from some responsibilities, but it is also your responsibility to face grief. Don't avoid it.

Preparations

Make a list of people to notify about the death. (Most people find the list easier to compose before the person dies.) Ideally, ask a friend or relative to make these calls for you. People may want to be with you at your side; however, it's your decision to make.

The list should include phone numbers for:
- the physician
- the medical school or society for the bequeathed body
- relatives
- friends
- pallbearers (if desired)
- the funeral director
- the decedent's attorney
- the decedent's employer

TIP: Bereavement air fares are discounted by 15% to 50% off full fares for passengers with a death in the family. Most flexible: TWA and Continental, which also offer discounts in cases of critical illness. Some hotels also offer special rates.

Notices For the death notice or obituary for the newspaper, make a list that includes the names of the deceased's:
- parents
- spouse or companion
- siblings
- children
- grandchildren (number only, not names)

Also include the individual's:
- birthplace
- educational background
- affiliation with professional organizations
- affiliation with community organizations

When death occurs

Death usually occurs peacefully. The family should have talked with their physician beforehand to learn what to expect in terms of time and characteristics. They should have discussed if, and under what conditions, they will call the paramedics.

Who to contact

After death has been determined by checking the pulse, there is no need to contact the police and coroner unless death occurred suddenly, or by violent or accidental means. Do contact the physician, funeral director and the clergy if they are not already there.

If death occurs without a physician in attendance, you'll need to make arrangements for a medical professional to provide a signed death certificate. The patient's physician, a home care nurse, or hospice staff member may legally sign the document, depending upon the state and county in which the death took place.

Immediate paperwork

- Ask for at least a dozen certified copies of the death certificate.

- Inform the Social Security Administration of the death.

Promptly consult an attorney to help with legal matters. Locate the will and letter of instruction. You may have difficulty in finding the deceased's will. If so, the best place to begin your search is in the decedent's personal files at home. Next, check with the decedent's attorney or banker, or the probate registrar. If you cannot find a will, you should see an attorney to learn if it is necessary to petition the probate court and request the appointment of an administrator over the estate. Note: small estates can be distributed without a will.

Disposition arrangements	• If a cemetery lot has already been purchased, locate the certificate. If not, and a lot is desired, purchase a lot or space in a cemetery, mausoleum or crypt. • Arrange a funeral or memorial service. (See Chapter 10 for final arrangements, also known as disposition.) • Arrange for an after-service luncheon or gathering, if one is desired. • Prepare for paperwork following the funeral or memorial service. (See Chapter 10.) • Other services are available by checking under the community services section in your phone directory for Death and Dying.

Disposition, Funerals, Cemeteries and Bereavement

"So, does it come in any other colors?"

This question was asked by a 9-year-old curious about caskets.

Note: The above attempt at humor is included to help offset an inescapably difficult subject.

Preparation

Planning is the best way to assure that whoever arranges a funeral or memorial service will handle it according to the wishes of the deceased. Putting final wishes in writing and discussing them with probable survivors will reduce their burden. Some people wish to have no ceremony at all. Other people want a ceremony to give survivors something on which to focus as 'something they can do'.

The emotional issues

Arranging a funeral is usually a very emotional task for survivors. They may be confused, disoriented, or numbed by shock. It is best to enlist the aid of a close friend to accompany you and help offset the pressures of guilt, time and unethical funeral directors.

First steps after a death

In a medical facility

A hospital or nursing home may hold the body for a short time. This allows you time to choose among several funeral homes or immediate disposition companies, according to price, experience or location. (An autopsy may be performed during this transition time, but an appropriate friend or family member must give approval or make the request.) The medical facility also may hold and transfer the body to the funeral home or crematorium for a fee. It will be necessary for a family member or friend to sign the document allowing relocation of the body.

At home	If death occurs at home, Chapter 9 explains which professionals—usually a certified physician— to call to provide a signed death certificate.
Away from home	If death occurs far from home, a funeral director or memorial society can arrange shipping, as well as other details. Death overseas or in other countries involves contacting the nearest American embassy or consulate to help make arrangements according to local regulations. The embassy or consulate will bill for the services, which may range from two hundred to several thousand dollars. For military personnel, the American Red Cross can be of help.

Disposition of the remains **Funeral homes**	Funeral homes typically present consumers with set-price packages. They offer convenience, but are usually the most costly method of disposition.
Crematoriums	Most crematoriums have facilities for holding small, brief commemorative services.
Direct-disposition companies	If you would like to avoid the use of a funeral home, cost-effective direct-disposition companies are available. They generally offer inexpensive, simple dispositions and completion of the necessary paperwork. They generally charge anywhere from $250 to $1,000. Look for them in the phone book yellow pages listed under Funeral Advisors. Some disposition companies advertise in the obituary pages of local newspapers.
Non-profit memorial societies	Non-profit memorial and funeral societies can refer consumers to cooperating funeral directors to obtain an inexpensive, but adequate, funeral or disposition. It is possible to arrange for a funeral and disposition without a funeral director.

Decisions to make	Depending upon personal preferences, religion, local custom and legal requirements, decisions should be based upon:

- type of final disposition (burial, cremation, entombment, donation to a research institution or organ bank, or other)
- type of ceremony (if any)
- cost
- the person selected to carry out the final arrangements

The previous four factors will help determine the following details.

Organ or research donation	Minimal costs are associated with the donation of the remains, but arrangements must be made in advance. The Living Bank (a registry of donors), the American Medial Association or groups such as the Eye Bank Association of America can coordinate the donation of specific organs. Donors must complete a Uniform Donor Card. UDC cards are available from various organizations listed in Chapters 9 and 11.

If the body is being donated, call the appropriate organization immediately upon death. Timely removal of donated organs is crucial for their use. For other types of disposition, you may call a funeral home or direct disposition company to pick up the remains.

Cremation	Cremation is often a less expensive alternative to other forms of disposition. The cost of cremation may include charges for the scattering or burial of the ashes. A container to transport the body is necessary for cremation; however, a casket is not required. Costs may range from $50 to $3,000.

Earth burial	An earth burial requires:

An earth burial requires:
- a casket
- a grave liner or vault (although these are not mandatory in all states)
- a plot
- a marker

Other services that you will be required to pay for include:
- a permit (depending upon local requirements)
- opening and closing the grave
- recording the burial in the cemetery's books
- cemetery upkeep

The type of casket selected can make the difference in cost between a $1,000 or $20,000 funeral. Ask for written price quotes and compare prices by phone. If an inexpensive casket is preferred, you must specifically ask to see them.

Embalming

Many funeral homes embalm whether or not the consumer has requested it. Some states require embalming only when death occurs from diseases such as cholera or bubonic plague, or when delays in burial occur. If a viewing of the body over several days is desired, embalming is probably necessary. If a closed casket viewing is selected, refrigeration may be all that is necessary. Make your decisions known.

Ceremonies

The funeral ceremony can range from a traditional funeral, with embalming, viewing and a religious service, to a simple memorial service or no service at all.

Some people forego a church service with the body present. Instead, they have a graveside service with family attending. They may later hold a memorial service for friends and family.

Public or private	Decide:

Public or private Decide:
- whether the funeral will be public or private
- where to hold the service
- who will officiate
- what music and readings will be used, if any
- whether the body will be present
- whether there will be a graveside service for the commitment of the body
- whether there will be an after-service luncheon or gathering for friends and relatives
- whether you wish memorial donations to be made to a specific organization
- whether you would like to donate excess flowers to a nursing home or some other organization after the service

Optional services Pay only for those services that you actually use. Of course, personal, religious and cultural beliefs will play a large part in decision-making. Products, services and issues to consider include:
- pallbearers
- hearse
- flower car
- transportation
- limousines
- motorcycle escort
- flowers
- instrumental music
- singing
- guest book
- acknowledgement cards
- prayer cards
- programs
- religious ritual
- readings
- films
- slides
- photographs

- tape recording
- nurse
- paperwork
- death notices and obituaries
- honoraria and gratuities

Paperwork

A funeral director can place the death notice in newspapers, obtain death certificates and file for death benefits; however, you can do these things yourself.

You will need many death certificates when applying for various benefits and gaining access to accounts. Be sure to order at least a dozen original death certificates from the attending medical physician, funeral director or the local government office that registers deaths. (It usually takes 30 days or more to get death certificates from the county compared to the 10 days it usually takes a mortuary to produce the documents.)

Payment

A funeral director may ask you, as the decision-maker, to guarantee payment by co-signing the funeral bill. If the costs exceed the estate's available benefits, you are accepting responsibility of payment by co-signing. In some cases, a 50% payment is requested immediately.

Paperwork following the funeral or memorial service

Because paperwork can become overwhelming, prepare a letter which states the decedent's name, birthdate, address and date of death. Make a number of copies, then add the applicable account number as a reference. This will save time and the emotional strain of re-writing the same type of letter.

Legal issues

- Obtain the decedent's original will, dates of birth and death, and Social Security number.
- Meet with an attorney to start probate, if applicable.
- Remove decedent's name as beneficiary of insurance policies.
- File a final tax return for the deceased for income earned in the year of death, if applicable.

Insurance claims	Notify and file claims with the appropriate insurance companies, memberships or organizations: • Auto insurance company • Clubs (such as American Automobile Association or fraternal organizations) • Credit card company (benefits may be payable as part of a group plan or membership privileges; and if used for ticket purchase, many credit cards provide life insurance automatically) • Credit union • Employer (disability and/or life insurance) • Personal insurance company (accident, disability, residence) • Medical insurance company • Mortgage company • Pension provider • Retirement fund • Social Security • Travel or trip insurance company • Union benefits • Veterans' Administration (burial benefits) • Worker's Compensation carrier
Financial institutions	Cancel and destroy credit cards, and notify: • Banks • Credit card and other charge account companies • Accountant/tax preparer • Stockbroker
Services	• Stop deliveries of newspapers and mail, or have mail rerouted to your address if you are handling the estate. • Notify utility companies, if applicable • Notify the Department of Motor Vehicles, if applicable.

	• Maintain or terminate agreements with rental or leasing agencies, membership plans, lodges or fraternal organizations, subscriptions and/or book clubs.
Thank-you notes	Maintain a list of the flowers, cards and donations that have been received. On the enclosure cards that arrive with the flowers, write the name of the sender and the type of remembrance sent (flowers, plant, etc.).

Additional reading

There are many books available to help you, your family and your friends through the bereavement process. A number of them are listed in Chapter 12.

It's Your Choice: The Practical Guide to Planning a Funeral
by Thomas C Nelson

Caring for Your Own Dead
by Lisa Carlson is another practical and informative book about alternative care.

Chapter 11

Organizations and other information sources

Probably the best source of information is an association whose purpose is to acquire and dispense knowledge about your particular illness. Other organizations may provide information regarding the availability of services and qualified professionals in your community.

For specific information for seniors, helpful information can be located in the senior services section of your phone book and County Office on Aging (found in the Government pages of the phone book). These resources can refer you to nursing facilities, programs for seniors, respite care workers and geriatric counselors specializing in helping families with aging relatives. Additional agencies can be found in the phone book yellow pages under the heading "Associations" or "Senior Citizens' Services & Organizations".

AAAs - Area Agency on Aging
More than 600 agencies across the nation. Find them in your phone book under "Aging" or public service listings.

ACTION
1100 Vermont Avenue, NW
Washington, DC 20525
(800) 424-8867
Federal agency that administers domestic volunteer programs, including Foster Grandparent Program, Senior Companion Program and others.

Administration on Aging (AoA)
Department of Health and Human
Services
330 Independence Avenue, SW
Washington, DC 20201
(202) 619-0724: general information
(202) 619-0641: publications

Aging Network Services
4400 East-West Highway, Suite 907
Bethesda, MD 20814
(301) 657-4329
Help with long-distance care-giving.

**Alzheimer's Association/ADRDA/
National**
360 N. Michigan Avenue, Suite 601
Chicago, IL 60601
(800) 621-0379

**Alzheimer's Disease Education and
Referral Center**
#NIAC, P.O. Box 8250
Silver Spring, Maryland 20907
(800) 438-4380

**American Association for
Acupuncture and Oriental Medicine**
1424 16th Street, NW, Suite 501
Washington, D.C. 20036
(202) 265-2287
Alternative treatments.

**American Association for Geriatric
Psychiatry**
P.O. Box 376A
Greenbelt, MD 20770
(301) 220-0952

**American Association of Homes
for the Aging**
901 E Street, N.W., Suite 500
Washington, DC 20004
(202) 783-2242
Represents not-for-profit nursing homes
and residential life care communities.

**American Association of Retired Persons
(AARP)**
601 E Street NW
Washington, DC 20049
(202) 434-2277

American Association of Suicidology
2459 South Ash Street
Denver, CO 80222
(303) 692-0985
A clearinghouse addressing aspects of
suicide, including the referral of survivors
of suicide to local resources.

American Board of Medical Specialties
1007 Church St., Suite 404
Evanston, IL 60201
(800) 776-2378

American Civil Liberties Union (ACLU)
132 West 43rd St.
New York, NY 10036
(202) 944-9800
Free publication list. National organization actively involved in the protection of
constitutional rights.

American Diabetes Association
1970 Chain Bridge Road
McLean, VA 22109-0512
(800) 232-3472

**American Foundation
for the Blind**
Product Center
100 Enterprise Place
P.O. Box 7044
Dover, DE 19903
(800) 829-0500

American Health Care Association
1201 L Street, N.W.
Washington, DC 20005
(202) 842-4444

American Heart Association
7272 Greenville Avenue
Dallas, Texas 75231-4599
(214) 706-1341- Fax
(214) 373-6300

American Heart Association's Stroke
Clubs of America
P.O. Box 15186
860 N. Highway 183
Austin, TX 78761

American Hospital Association
Division of Ambulatory Care
840 North Lake Shore Drive
Chicago, IL 60611
(312) 280-6216

American Kidney Fund
6110 Executive Boulevard, Suite 110
Rockville, Maryland 20852
(800) 638-8299

American Lung Association
1740 Broadway
New York, NY 10019
(212) 315-8700

American Occupational Therapy
Association
1383 Picard Drive
Rockville, MD 20850

American Osteopathic Association
142 E. Ontario
Chicago, IL 60611
(312) 280-5800

American Parkinson Disease Association
60 Bay Street
Staten Island, NY 10301
(800) 223-2732

American Physical Therapy Association
1740 Broadway
New York, NY 10019

American Society for Clinical Hypnosis
2400 East Devon Ave., Suite 218
Des Plaines, Illinois 60018
(708) 297-3317
Hypnosis for people with chronic pain to
learn helpful deep relaxation techniques.

American Society on Aging
(800) 537-9728

American Speech-Language-Hearing
Association
10801 Rockville Pike
Rockville, MD 20852
(301) 897-5700
(800) 638-8255 (Consumer Helpline)

ASK-A-NURSE Connection
An information and referral service that
connects you to knowledgeable registered
nurses.
(800) 535-1111
The 24-hour automated service will provide you with the phone number of the
nearest ASK-A-NURSE connection.

Association for Applied Psychophysiology
and Biofeedback
10200 W. 44th Avenue, Suite 304
Wheat Ridge, Colorado 80033
(303) 422-8436
Some cancer patients have found biofeedback helpful as an addition to other pain
control techniques or medications.

Association for Brain Tumor Research
3725 North Talman Avenue
Chicago, Illinois 60618
(312) 286-5571

Association for the Care of Children's Health
7910 Woodmont Avenue, Suite 300
Bethesda, MD 20814
(301) 654-6549
A clearinghouse for information concerning children with chronic or terminal illnesses. Offers publications with practical advice.

Association of Rehabilitation Facilities
5530 Wisconsin Avenue, NW
Washington, DC 20015

Bereavement and Loss Center of New York
170 E. 83 St.
New York, NY 10028
(212) 879-5655

Cancer Care, Inc.
1180 Avenue of the Americas
New York, New York 10036
(212) 221-3300

Cancer Hotline
(800) 525-3777

Cancer Information Service
(800) 638-6694 National office

Candlelighters Childhood Cancer Foundation
1901 Pennyslvania Ave., Suite 1001
Washington, DC 20006
(202) 659-5136

CanSurmount and I Can Cope
Sponsored by the American Cancer Society
1599 Clifton Rd. NE
Atlanta, GA 30329
(404) 320-3333

Caregiver Assistance Program
Long Term Care Unit
New York State Office for the Aging
Two Empire State Plaza
Albany, New York 12223-0001
(518) 474-8388

Catholic Golden Age
400 Lackawanna Avenue
Scranton, PA 18505
(717) 342-3294

Children of Aging Parents (CAPS)
Woodbourne Office Campus
Suite 302-A
1609 Woodbourne Road
Levittown, PA 19057
(215) 945-6900
Enclose $1 and a self-addressed stamped envelope with any request for brochures or information.

Children's Hospice International
901 N. Washington Street, Suite 700
Alexandria, VA 22314
(800) 242-4453

Choice in Dying
200 Varick Street
New York, NY 10014
(212) 366-5540

Closing the Gap
P.O. Box 68
Henderson, MN 56044
(612) 248-3294
Specializes in computer technology for special education and rehabilitation.

Commission on Legal Problems of the Elderly
American Bar Association
1800 M Street, NW
Washington, DC 20036
(202) 331-2297

Compassionate Friends
P.O. Box 3696
Oak Brook, Il 60522-3696
(708) 990-0010   Fax- (708) 990-0246
Send a SASE to learn about this support
organization. $1 will help defray costs.

**Concern for Dying/Society for
the Right to Die**
250 West 57th Street
New York, NY 10107
(212) 246-6962 or (212) 246-6973

**Continuing Care Accreditation
Commission**
1129 20th Street, NW
Washington, DC 20036
(202) 828-9439
Can provide a list of accredited facilities.

Corporate Angel Network
Building One
Westchester Airport
White Plains, New York 10604
(914) 328-1313
Organization helps arrange free trans-
portation to and from distant treatment
centers using corporate aircraft that have
empty seats during business trips.
Financial need is not a requirement.

Counseling for Caregivers
(215) 455-6320

**Department of Heath and Human
Services**
Social Security Administration
Baltimore, Maryland 21235

Direct Link for the Disabled
(805) 688-1603
Addresses medical, social, financial and
work-related issues for the disabled.

Eldercare Locator
(800) 677-1116
An agency to help identify community
resources for seniors. Have the following
ready when you call: name, address and zip
code of the person you are helping and
type of assistance sought.

Elderhostel
100 Boylston Street
Boston, Massachusetts 02116
Provides week-long educational
experiences for people 60+ years.

Elder Links
2032 E. Monterey Way
Phoenix, AZ 85016
(602) 957-4883
Geriatric care managers.

Encyclopedia of Associations
-found in the reference section of your
library

Families of Nursing Home Residents
(415) 682-8330

Family Survival Project
(415) 434-3388
(800) 445-8106

**Friends and Relatives of the
Institutionalized Aged**
11 John Street
New York, NY 10038
(212) 732-4455

**Foundation for Hospice
and Home Care**
519 C Street, N.E.
Washington, DC 20002
(202) 547-6586

Gray Panthers
2025 Pennsylvania Avenue, NW
Suite 821
Washington, DC 20006
(202) 466-3132

Health Insurance Association of America
National Insurance Consumer Helpline
1025 Connecticut Avenue, NW, Suite 1200
Washington, DC 20036
(202) 223-7780
(800) 942-4242 Hotline

Help for Incontinent People
P.O. Box 544
Union, SC 29379
(803) 864-3913

Hemlock Society
(310) 476-8696

Hospice Association of America
519 C Street, NE
Washington, DC 20002
(202) 547-7424

Hospice Education Institute
5 Essex Square, Suite 3-B
Essex, CT 06426
(800) 331-1620

Humor Project, Inc.
Dept. CR
110 Spring Street
Saratoga Springs, NY 12866
Write for free information on books and
magazines that address the positive healing
power of humor. Send a self-addressed
envelope with 75 cents postage.

Institute of Certified Financial Planners
7600 E. Eastman Avenue, Suite 301
Denver, CO 80231
(800) 282-7526

International Association of
Laryngectomees
American Cancer Society
(404) 329-7651
Support programs for people who have
lost their voice as a result of cancer.

International Pain Foundation
909 N.E. 43rd St., Suite 306
Seattle, WA 98105-6020

JASA/Jewish Association for Services for
the Aged
40 W. 68th St.
New York, NY 10023
(212) 724-3200

Joint Commission for
Accreditation of Health Care
Organizations
875 North Michigan Avenue
Chicago, IL 60611
(302) 642-6061

Legal Counsel for the Elderly
P.O. Box 96474
Washington, DC 20090-6474

Legal Counsel for the Elderly
American Association of Retired Persons
1331 H Street, NW, Suite 10005
Washington, DC 20005
(202) 234-0970

Leukemia Society of America
733 Third Avenue
New York, NY 10017
(212) 573-8484

Lupus Foundation of America
8420 Delmar
St. Louis, MO 63124
(314) 432-0008

Make Today Count, Inc.
168 Panoramic
Camdenton, MO 65065
(314) 346-6644
Support group for people with life-
threatening illnesses.

Medicare Information Hotline
U.S. Department of Health and Human
Services
Health Care Financing Administration
Washington, DC 20201
(000) 888-1770 Recorded message
(800) 888-1998 To request written
material or information.

Medicare Medigap Insurance Fraud Line
U.S.Department of Health and Human
Services
Health Care Financing Administration
Washington, DC 20201
(800) 638-6833

Mended Hearts
c/o American Heart Association
7320 Greenville Ave.
Dallas, TX 75231
(214) 706-1442
Support group for heart disease patients
and their families.

Modern Talking Picture Service
5000 Park Street North
St. Petersburg, FL 33709
(800) 237-6213
They will mail a catalog of 3,000 captioned
films for hearing-impaired people.

**National Academy of Elder Law
Attorneys, Inc.**
655 N. Alvernon Way, Suite 108
Tucson, Arizona 85711
(602) 881-4005
Send a SASE to request their free pamphlet
*Questions & Answers When Looking for an
Elder Law Attorney*

**National AIDS Information
Clearinghouse**
P.O. Box 6003
Rockville, MD 20849-6003
(800) 458-5231

**National Alliance of Breast Cancer
Organizations**
1180 Avenue of the Americas
New York, New York 10036
(212) 719-0154

National Association for Home Care
519 C Street, NE
Washington, DC 20002
(202) 547-7424

**National Association of Area Agencies on
Aging**
1112-16th Street, NW
Washington, DC 20036
(202) 296-8130
(800) 677-1116 Eldercare Locator
A social services long-distance referral
agency.

**National Association of Health
Underwriters**
1000 Connecticut Ave., NW, Suite 1111
Washington, DC 20036

National Association for Home Care
519 C Street, N.E.
Stanton Park
Washington, DC 20002
(202) 547-7424

**National Association of Private Geriatric
Care Managers**
655 N. Alvernon
Suite 108
Tucson, AZ 85711
(602) 881-8008
Send a SASE for a free referral to a local
geriatric-care manager.

**National Association for the Visually
Handicapped**
22 W. 21st Street
New York, NY 10010
(212) 889-3141

National Association of Insurance
Commissioners
1125 Grand Ave.
Kansas City, MO 64106

National Association of Meal Programs
Box 6344
604 West North Avenue
Pittsburgh, PA 15212

National Association of Private Geriatric
Care Managers
655 N. Alvernon Way, Suite 108
Tucson, AZ 85711
(602) 881-8008
Ask for a list of care managers in your state
and the state of the care receiver.

National Cancer Care Foundation
1180 Avenue of the Americas
New York, NY 10036
(212) 221-3300

National Cancer Institute
(800) 422-6237

National Center for the Black Aged
1424 K Street, NW
Suite 500
Washington, DC 20005
(202) 637-8400

National Center for Home Equity
Conversion
1210 East College Drive, Suite 300
Marshall, MN 56258
(507) 532-323
Send a SASE and $1 for their 'Reverse
Mortgage Locator'.

National Citizen's Coalition for Nursing
Home Reform
1224 M Street, NW, Suite 301
Washington, DC 20005
(202) 393-2018

National Coalition for Cancer
Survivorship
323 8th St, SW
Alburquerque, NM 87102
(505) 764-9956

National Consumers League
815 15th Street, NW, Suite 928
Washington, DC 20005
(202) 639-8140

National Council of Senior Citizens
925 15th Street, NW
Washington, DC 20005
(202) 624-9500

National Head Injury Foundation
1776 Massachusetts Avenue, NW,
Suite 100
Washington, DC 20036
(800) 444-6443

National Heart, Lung and Blood Institute
(301) 951-3260

National Home Caring Council
519 C Street, NE
Washington, DC 20002
(202) 547-6586

National Hospice Organization
1901 North Moore St., Suite 901
Arlington, VA 22209
(800) 658-8898

National Information Center on Deafness
Gallaudet University
800 Florida Avenue N.E.
Washington, DC 20002
(202) 651-5051

National Institute on Adult Day Care
The National Council on the Aging
409 3rd St. SW
Washington, DC 20024
(202) 479-1200

National Institute of Allergy and
Infectious Diseases
(800) 342-2437 AIDS Hotline

National Institute of Arthritis and
Musculoskeletal and Skin Diseases
(301) 495-4484

National Institute of Diabetes and
Digestive and Kidney Diseases
(301) 468-2162 Diabetes
(301) 468-6344 Digestive Diseases
(301) 468-6345 Kidneys and Urology

National Institutes of Health
Building #31
Room 2B03
Bethesda, MD 20892
Request their list of NIH publications.

National Institute of Mental Health
(800) 421-4211

National Institute of Neurological
Disorders and Stroke
(800) 352-9424 - general information
(800) 438-4380 - Alzheimer's Disease

National Insurance Consumer Helpline
(800) 942-4242

National Insurance Consumer
Organization (NICO)
121 N. Payne St.
Alexandria, Virginia 22314
(703) 549-8050

National League for Nursing
350 Hudson St.
New York, NY 10014
(212) 989-9393

National Organization for Rare Disorders
P.O. Box 8923
New Fairfield, CT 06812-1783
(800) 999-6673

National Rehabilitation and Information
Center/ABLE DATA
8455 Colesville Road, Suite 935
Silver Spring, MD 20910
(800) 346-2742

National Senior Citizens Law Center
2025 M Street, NW, Suite 400
Washington, DC 20036
(202) 887-5280

National Shared Housing Resource Center
431 Pine St.
Burlington, Vermont 05401
(802) 862-2727

National Stroke Association
300 E. Hampden Ave., Suite 240
Englewood, CO 80110-2654
(303) 762-9922

National Volunteer Agency
ACTION
The Senior Companion Program
Washington, DC 20525

Nurses of America
New York, NY
(212) 989-9393

Office of Disease Prevention and Health
Promotion
National Health Information Center
P.O. Box 1133
Washington, DC 20013-1133
(800) 336-4797
Provides 800-numbers offering a range of
services, referrals and written materials.

Older Women's League
666 11th St., SW
Suite 700
Washington, DC 20001
(202) 783-6686

Organ Donor Hotline
United Network for Organ Sharing
1100 Boulders Parkway, Suite 500
P.O. Box 13770
Richmond, VA 23225-8770
(800) 243-6667

People with AIDS Coalition
(800) 828-3280

People's Medical Society
462 Walnut Street
Allentown, PA 18102
(800) 624-8773
For $15 membership fee, they can de-code your hospital bill.

Public Citizen Health Research Group
2000 P St. NW
Washington, DC 20036
Lists United States doctors disciplined by state medical boards.

Reach to Recovery
c/o American Cancer Society
1599 Clifton Rd. NE
Atlanta, GA 30329
(404) 320-3333

Safe Return
A 24-hour 800-number service to call when a person with Alzheimer's disease is missing. $25 registration.
(800) 272-3900

Senior Information and Referral Services, Inc.
(800) 255-9333

Simon Foundation for Continence
P.O. Box 815
Wilmette, IL 6009
(800) 237-4666

Social Security Administration (SSA)
Office of Public Inquiries
6401 Security Boulevard
Baltimore, Maryland 21235
(800) 772-1213 or (301) 965-1234

Society for the Advancement of Travel for the Handicapped
347 5th Avenue, Suite 610
New York, NY 10016
(212) 447-7284

Society for the Right to Die
250 W. 57th St.
New York, N.Y. 10107
(212) 586-6248 - fax(212) 246-6973

Society of Real Estate Appraisers
645 N. Michigan Ave.
Chicago, IL 60611
Request free copy of the national directory of designated appraisers.

Stroke Connection
American Heart Association
7272 Greenville Ave.
Dallas, TX 75231
(214) 373-6300

Stroke Foundation
898 Park Ave.
New York, NY 10021
(212) 734-3461

Summer Camps for Children with Cancer
(800) 227-2345

Survivors of Suicide
Suicide Prevention Center, Inc.
P.O. Box 1393
Dayton, OH 45401-1393
(513) 223-9096

Touchstone Support Network
378 Cambridge Avenue, Suite K
Palo Alto, CA 94306
(415) 328-4495

United Network for Organ Sharing (UNOS)
Box 13770
Richmond, VA 23225
(800) 243-6667

United Ostomy Association
36 Executive Park, Suite 120
Irvine, CA 92714
(714) 660-8624

United Seniors Health Cooperative
Dept. J
1331 H Street NW, Suite 500
Washington, DC 20005
Send a check for $2.75 to receive Medicare and Medigap update reports.

Veterans' Association
(800) 827-1000

Veterans' Legal Services Project
Washington, D.C.
(202) 265-8305

We Can Do
1800 Augusta, Suite 150
Houston, TX 77057
(713) 780-1057

Wellness Community
2190 Colorado Avenue
Santa Monica, CA 90404-3503
(310) 453-2300
Cancer support group.

Woman's Financial Information Program
Educational program available thru AARP (American Association of Retired Persons) to help women take charge of their financial lives.
(202) 434-2277

WORLD: Women Organized to Respond to Life-Threatening Diseases
(510) 658-6930

World Institute on Disability
(510) 763-4100

WPS Directory of Services for the Widowed in the United States and Canada
To receive a free directory of national/local groups, send a postcard to:
WPS (Widowed Persons Services)
AARP (American Association of Retired Persons)
1909 K Street, NW
Washington, DC 20049
(202) 728-4370

Y-ME National Organization for Breast Cancer
Information and Support
18220 Harwood Ave
Homewood, IL 60430
(708) 799-8338

Chapter 12

Publications and Books

The following is a list of suggested resources. The publications can be found or ordered through bookstores, or requested from specific addresses as noted. Some of the publications are free if you send a SASE (self-addressed stamped envelope). Many of the books are available in libraries.

Individual drug companies often prepare excellent short booklets providing very useful information about the nature of the medication and proper treatment of your illness. You can get the pharmaceutical company's address from your doctor to request the information.

AARP Books (American Association of Retired Persons)
1. Before You Buy: A Guide to Long-Term-Care Insurance

2. Caregiving
$13.95 (AARP Members $9.95)

3. Essential Guide to Wills, Estates, Trusts and Death Taxes
$12.95 (AARP Members $9.95)

4. It's Your Choice: A Practical Guide to Planning a Funeral
$4.95 (AARP members $3.00)

5. Miles Away and Still Caring: A Guide for Long Distance Caregivers

6. Staying at Home: A Guide to Long-Term Care & Housing

7. The Gadget Book
$10.95 (AARP members $7.95)

8. The Nursing Home Handbook
$9.95 (AARP members $6.95)

To order the above books, write: AARP Books; Scott, Foresman and Company, 1865 Miner Street, Des Plaines, IL 60016. Add $1.75 per total order (NOT per book) for shipping and handling.

A Checklist of Concerns/Resources for Caregivers
Excellent free pamphlet from AARP
(202) 434-2277

A Comprehensive Guide to Medicare and Health Insurance for Older People
by Dale M. Larson; LTC, Inc.
10940 Northeast 33rd Place, Suite 205
Bellevue, WA 98004
$9.95

Aging and Our Families: Handbook for Family Caregivers
by Donna Couper

Aging and the Law
by Peter Strauss

A Guide for the Donation of Organs and Tissues for Transplantation
United Network for Organ Sharing
Box 13770
Richmond, VA 23225

A Guide to Choosing Medicare Supplemental Insurance
United Seniors Health Cooperative
1334 G Street NW
Washington, DC 20005

AIDS: The Ultimate Challenge
by Elisabeth Kubler-Ross

Alternatives to Nursing Homes
Free, send a SASE to:
Bottom Line/Persona
Box 579
Springfield, New Jersey 07081

Alzheimer's: A Caregiver's Guide and Sourcebook
by Howard Gruetzner

American Cancer Society Cancer Book
The American Cancer Society

A Path with Heart
by Jack Kornfield

A Second Start: A Widow's Guide to Financial Survival at a Time of Emotional Crisis
by Judith N. Brown and Christina Baldwin

Answers
Magazine published for adult children of aging parents.
Subscription: $15
201 Tamal Vista Blvd.
Corte Madera, CA 94925-9800
(415) 924-4737

Avoiding the Medicaid Trap: How to Beat the Catastrophic Cost of Nursing Home Care
by Armond Budish

Beat the Nursing Home Trap
by Joseph Matthews

Before You Buy: A Guide to Long-term Care Insurance
Free from:
The American Association of Retired Persons (AARP)
1909 K Street NW
Washington, DC 20049

Before You Call the Doctor: Safe, Effective Self-Care for Over 300 Common Medical Problems
by Ann Simons, M.D., Bobbie Hasselbring, and Michael Castleman

Being a Widow
by Lynn Caine

Bereavement: A Magazine of Hope and Healing
Bereavement Publishing
350 Gradle Drive
Carmel, IN 46032
(317) 846-9429

Beyond Endurance: When a Child Dies
by Ronald J. Knapp

Cancer Information: Where to Find Help
AICR (American Institute for Cancer
Research) free booklet, write to:
AICR National Headquarters
Washington, DC 20069

Care-Giving
by Jo Horne

*Care Management: Arranging for Long
Term Care*
Free booklet from:
AARP Fulfillment (D13803)
P.O. Box 22796
Long Beach, CA 90801-5796

*Caring for an Aging Parent: Have I Done
All I Can?*
by Jane Avis Ball

*Choices: Realistic Alternatives in Cancer
Treatment*
by Marion Morra and Eve Potts

*Coming Home: A Guide to Dying at Home
with Dignity*
by Deborah Duda

*Concerning Death: A Practical Guide for
the Living*
by Earl Grollman

Coping with the Loss of a Pet
by Christina M. Lemieux, Ph.D.

*Daughters of the Elderly: Building
Partnerships in Caregiving*
by J. Norris.
Indiana University Press. $9.95

Depression Guidelines
Dept. AL
P.O. Box 8547
Silver Spring, MD 20907
Free from the U.S. Public Health Service
Agency for Health Care Policy and
Research
Send a postcard to request their free
brochure.

Do Yourself Justice
American Association of Retired Persons
(AARP)
AARP Fulfillment
1909 K St. NW
Washington, DC 20049
Free publication.

*Drivers 55 Plus: Test Your Own
Performance*
AAA Foundation for Traffic Safety
1730 M St., NW, Suite 401
Washington, DC 20036
(American Automobile
Association)
Free self-rating form.

Dying: Facing the Facts
by Wass, Berardo, and Neimeyer
A textbook which includes discussion of
death anxiety.

*Easing the Passage: A Guide for
Prearranging and Ensuring a Pain-Free
and Tranquil Death via a Living Will,
Personal Medical Mandate, and Other
Medical, Legal, and Ethical Resources*
by David E. Outerbridget and Alan R.
Hersh, M.D.
A good gift for skeptical parents.

*Elder Care: Choosing & Financing Long-
Term Care*
by Joseph Matthews, Nolo Press

Elder Care: Coping with Late-Life Crisis
by James Kenny, Ph.D. and Stephen
Spicer, M.D.

Eldercare in the '90s
by Friends and Relatives of the
Institutionalized Aged
(212) 732-4455

*Everything Your Heirs Need to Know:
Your Assets, Family History and Final
Wishes*
by David S. Magee
A book, with cleverly designed forms and
document pockets, that might make a
good gift for your parents.

*Exemptions, Standard Deductions and
Filing Information*
Free IRS publication #501:
How to claim a parent as a dependent.
To order; call (800) 829-3676

Facing Death
by Robert E. Kavanaugh

*Family Guide to Wills, Funerals & Estate
Planning: How to Protect Yourself and
Your Survivors*
by Theodore E. Hughes and David Klein

*Final Passages: Positive Choices for the
Dying and Their Loved Ones*
by Judith Ahronheim, M.D., and Doron
Weber

Health Care Powers of Attorney
Free booklet available by sending a post-
card with your address to:
AARP Fulfillment
(Stock No. D13895)
1909 K Street, NW
Washington, D.C. 20049

*Home Care for Seriously Ill Children: A
Manual for Parents*
published by Children's Hospice
International
(800) 242-4453 (703) 684-0330

*Home Care for the Elderly: A Complete
Guide*
by Jay Portnow, M.D., with Martha
Houtmann, R.N.

*Home Health Care Solution: A Complete
Consumer Guide*
by Janet Zhun Nassif

Hospice Handbook
by Larry Beresford

*How to Care for Your Aging Parents... and
still have a life of your own!*
by J. Michael Dolan

*How to Care for Your Parents: A
Handbook for Adult Children*
by Nora Jean Levi
Storm King Press
P.O. Box 2089,
Friday Harbor, WA 98250
(206) 378-3910

How to Donate the Body or Its Organs
Free. Request Publication No.
(NIH) 79-776
U.S. Department of Health and
Human Services
Washington, D.C.

*How to Talk to Your Doctor: The
Questions to Ask*
by Janet R. Maurer. 1986. Simon &
Schuster. Out of print book; however,
found in many city libraries.

*"I Don't Know What to Say..." How to
Help and Support Someone Who Is Dying*
by Robert Buckman

*It's Your Choice: A Consumer's Guide to
Planning a Funeral (804)*
Free from:
AARP
1909 K Street, NW
Washington, DC 20049

*Keeping Family Stories Alive: A Creative
Guide to Taping Your Family Life and Lore*
by Vera Rosenbluth

Keys to Planning for Long-Term Custodial Care
by David Ness

Let the Patient Decide
by Louis S. Baer, M.D.

Living Beyond Limits: New Hope and Help for Facing Life-Threatening Illness
by David Spiegel, M.D.

Living Longer, Living Better: Adventures in Community Housing forThose in the Second Half of Life
by Jane Porcino, Ph.D.

Living When a Loved One Has Died
by Earl A. Grollman

Living Wills and More
by Terry J. Barnett

Long Distance Caregiving: A Survival Guide for Faraway Caregivers
by Angela Heath

Long-Term Care: A Dollar and Sense Guide
Available from The United Seniors Health Cooperative
1331 H St. NW, Suite 500
Washington, DC 20005-4706
$10.00

Making Medical Decisions: How to Make Difficult Medical and Ethical Choices for Yourself and Your Family
by Thomas Scully, M.D., and Celia Scully

Making Peace with Your Parents: The Key to Enriching Your Life and All Your Relationships
by Harold H. Bloomfield, M.D., with Leonard Felder, Ph.D.

Managing Medications
Free brochure. Send a SASE with your request to:
Dept. S
P.O. Box 15329
Stamford, CT 06901

Managing Your Health Care Finances
published by United Seniors Health Cooperative
Send your $10 check made out to:
USHC
1331 H Street NW, Suite 500
Washington, DC 20005-4706.

Medicaid Planning Handbook
by Alexander A. Bove, Jr.

Medical Directive/Harvard Health Letter
P.O. Box 380
Boston, MA 02117
(617) 432-1485
Pamphlet describes typical situations when advance directives may be necessary, plus a place to document your wishes should you face similar situations.
For 2 copies, send $5.00 and a self-addressed, stamped envelope.

Medicare Made Easy
Available from People's Medical Society
462 Walnut St.
Allentown, PA 18102
(800) 624-8773

Medicare, Medigap, Catastrophic Care and You
by Randy Freudig
R.A. Freudig Associates
P.O. Box D, Warrington, PA 18976
$17.00

No Lifetime Guarantee: Dealing with the Details of Death
by Katie Maxwell

Nutrition and the Cancer Patient
by Joyce Daly Margie and Abby S. Bloch,
M.S., R.D.

Nutrition for the Chemotherapy Patient
by Janet Ramstack and Ernest Rosenbaum,
M.D.

Nutrition for the Cancer Patient
by Jane Bradley and Susan Nass

Office of Public Affairs, SSA
Distribution Center
P.O. Box 17743
Baltimore, MD 21235
(310) 965-1720
Send for catalog listing the free Social
Security publications found at your local
SSA office.

Our Older Friends: A Guide for Visitors
by Joel T. Keys

Overcoming Your Grief
by Donald W. Steele

Parent Care Newsletter
Gerontology Center
University of Kansas
Lawrence, KS 66045

*Parent Care Survival Guide: Helping Your
Folks Through the Not-So-Golden Years*
by Enid Pritikin and Trudy Reece

Center for the Study of Aging
1331 H St. NW
Washington, DC 20005
$8.95 + $2.00

Planning for Incapacity: A Self-Help Guide
Send a check or money order for $5.00 per
book. Include your name,address and the
state(s) in which you are interested.

Plan Your Estate
by Denis Clifford, attorney

*Policy Wise: The Practical Guide
to Insurance Decisions for
Older Consumers (803)*
Free from: AARP
1909 K Street, NW
Washington, DC 20049

Questions and Answers about Pain Control
Request this free pamphlet from
Cancer Information Service
(800) 422-6237

*Questions and Answers When Looking for
An Elder Law Attorney*
National Academy of Elder Law Attorneys
655 N. Alvernon Way
Tucson, Arizona 85711
Include a SASE with your request.

Recovering from the Loss of a Sibling
by Katherine Fair Donnelly

Recovery From Bereavement
by Colin Murray Parkes, M.D., and Robert
Stuart Weiss, Ph.D.

Silent Grief: Living in the Wake of Suicide
by Christopher Lucas and Henry M.
Seiden

*Simple Will Book: How to Prepare a
Legally Valid Will*
Nolo Press

*Social Security Administration's free
publications available from:*
Department of Health and Human
Services
Social Security Administration
Baltimore, Maryland 21235

1) *Disability*- A guide to Social Security
disability benefits Medicare

2) *Retirement*- A guide to Social Security
retirement benefits

3) *Supplemental Security Income*- A guide
to the SSI program

4) *Survivors*- A guide to Social Security survivors benefits

5) *Understanding Social Security*- A brief overview of each of the Social Security programs

Suddenly Alone: A Woman's Guide to Widowhood
by Philomene Gates

Survival Handbook for Widows (and for Relatives and Friends Who Want to Understand)
by Ruth Jean Loewinsohn

Take Care! A Guide for Caregivers on How to Improve Their Self Care
Available from:
Amherst H. Wilder Foundation
919 Lafond Avenue
St. Paul, MN 55104
(612) 642-4060
$2.50

Talking With Your Aging Parents
by Mark A. Edinberg

Talking Books are available from the National Library Service for the Blind and Physically Handicapped Library of Congress
Washington, DC 20542
Ask for the free brochure *"Reading is for Everyone"*

The 36-Hour Day(a guide for caregivers)
by Nancy Mace and Peter Rabins

The Best Medicine: How to Choose the Top Doctors,the Top Hospitals, and the Top Treatments
by Robert Arnot, M.D.

The Big Squeeze: Balancing the Needs of Aging Parents, Dependent Children, and YOU
by Barbara A. Shapiro

The Caregiving Years: Advice for Children of Aging Parents
by Kirstin Lund and Mary McKeown Darts
60 East Marien West
St. Paul, MN 55118
$3.00

The Complete & Easy Guide to Social Security and Medicare
by Faustin F. Jehle
(800) 234-8791
$10.95

The Complete Guide to Long-Term Care
Phillips Publishing, Inc.
7811 Montrose Road
Potomac, MD 20854
(800) 777-5005
$43.95

Coping with Caregiving
by Vicki Schmall and Ruth Steihl

The Caregiver
Newsletter of the Duke Family Support Program.
The Caregiver
Box 3600 DUMC
Durham, NC 27710
$10/year subscription.

The Complete Book of Wills & Estates
by Henry Holt and Co.

The Courage to Grieve
by Judy Tatelbaum

The Encyclopedia of Estate Planning
Boardroom Classics
Box 736
Springfield, NJ 07081
Robert Holzman
$29.95

The Executor's Manual: Everything You Need to Know to Handle an Estate
by Charles K. Plotnick and Stephen R. Leimberg

The Nursing Home and You: Partners in Caring for a Relative with Alzheimer's Disease
Available from Triad Alzheimer's Association
P.O. Box 15622
Winston-Salem, NC 27113
$4.50 32-page paperback

The Nursing Home Experience: A Family Guide to Making It Better
by Marylou Hughes

The Path Through Grief: A Practical Guide
by Marguerite Bouvard with Evelyn Gladu

The People's Book of Medical Tests
by David S. Sobel, M.D., and Tom Ferguson, M.D.

The Power of Attorney Book
by Denis Clifford, Nolo Press

The Road Ahead: A Stroke Recovery Guide
Order from: National Stroke Association
300 E. Hampden Ave., Suite 240
Englewood, CO 80110-2654
(303) 762-9922
$16.50

The Second 50 Years- a reference manual for Senior Citizens
by Walter Cheney, William Diehm and Frank E. Seeley

The Simple Will Book
by Denis Clifford

The Loneliness of the Dying
by Edmund Jephcott

The Patient's Advocate: the Complete Handbook of Patient Rights
by B. Huttmann

Time to Care, Help for the Caregiver; Caregiver's Practical Help; Coping with Alzheimer's Disease
For a free copy of any of the 3 publications, write:
New York State Office for the Aging
Informal Caregiver's Project
2 Empire State Plaza
Albany, NY 12223-0001

To Be Old and Sad: Understanding Depression in the Elderly
by Nathan Billig, M.D.

Tomorrow's Choices
Free. AARP Fulfillment
1909 K Street, NW
Washington, DC 20049

Too Old to Cry... Too Young to Die
by Edith Pendleton

The Widow's Handbook: A Guide for Living
by Charlotte Fochner and Carol Cozart

Understanding Living Trusts
by Vickie Schumacher and Jim Schumacher

Understanding Long-Term Care Insurance
by Max E. Lemberger
National Association of Health Underwriters
1000 Connecticut Ave., NW, Suite 1111
Washington, DC 20036

Values History
Institute of Public Law
1117 Stanford, NE
Albuquerque, NM 87135
(505) 277-5006
Send check for $3.00 for nonlegal document that suggests topics to consider when completing an advance directive.

What You Need to Know About Cancer
Available from the Cancer Information
Service
(800) 422-6237

When Bad Things Happen to Good People
by Harold Kushner

*When Love Gets Tough: The Nursing
Home Decision*
by Doug Manning.
In-Sight Books, Inc., Drawer 2058
Hereford, TX 79045
$4.50 + postage

When Parents Die: A Guide for Adults
by Edward Myers

When Someone You Know Has AIDS
by Leonard J. Martelli

When Your Loved One is Dying
by E.A. Grollman

Who? What? Where?
A free booklet about senior women's
health & social issues.
For a copy, call:
National Institute on Aging
(800) 222-2225

Widow's Handbook: A Guide for Living
by Charlotte Foehner and Carol Cozart

Widow to Widow
by Phyllis Silverman

Will Organizer
Free booklet from American Institute for
Cancer Research
(202) 328-7744

You and Your Aging Parent
by Silverstone & Hyman

You Don't Have to Suffer
by Judy Tatelbaum

Your Aging Parents
by John Deedy

*Your Best is Good Enough: Aging Parents
and Your Emotions*
by V.E. Greenberg. Lexington Books.

The following free pamphlets discuss
aspects of childhood death. Send your
request to the address below and include a
self-addressed stamped envelope.

1. *Understanding Grief*

2. *Surviving Your Child's Suicide*

3. *Caring for Surviving Children*

4. *When a Child Dies*

5. *The Grief of Stepparents*

6. *How Can I Help?*

7. *Suggestions for Teachers and School
   Counselors*
The Compassionate Friends
P.O. Box 3696
Oak Brook, IL 60522-3696
(708) 990-0010 FAX (708) 990-0246

For young children
Grampa Doesn't Know It's Me
by Donna Guthrie. Alzheimer's Disease.

My Grandpa Died Today
by Joan Fassler

Nana Upstairs and Nana Downstairs
by Tomie DePaola

Chapter 13

Various Resources: Audio and video tapes, computer software and forms to order

Audio tapes

Solving the Retirement Puzzle
$19.95
Retirement Planning Associates
(800) 546-5406

Care givers

A Friend in Need: Caring for an Incapacitated Adult
video tape: $18.50
Council on Aging for Friend of the Court Conservator
COA for FCC
2115 The Alameda
San Jose, CA 95126

What Every Caregiver Ought to Know
Commerce Clearing House, Inc.
Cash Item Department
$5.00 paperback book
4025 W. Peterson Ave.
Chicago, IL 60646
(800) 248-3248

Gifts

A Loving Voice: A Caregiver's Book of Read-Aloud Stories for the Elderly
by Carolyn Banks & Janis Rizzo

Modern Talking Picture Service
15000 Park St. North
St. Petersburg, FL 33709
(800) 237-6213
Free catalog of 3,000 captioned films for hearing-impaired people.

Radio Memories
For a list of available cassettes, call
(914) 245-6609.

Talking Books
Available through the mail from the Library of Congress and its branch offices.

Positive Moves by Angela Lansbury
45-minute video tape includes gentle strength and stretching exercises, plus recipes and general tips for active living.
$19.95

Laughter Therapy
Allen Funt Productions
2359 Nichols Canyon Road
Los Angeles, CA 90046

Don't forget humor as a healing force.
Receive a 1-month free rental of old Candid Camera shows on videocassette by writing to the address above.

Health

Image Paths, Inc.
Box 5714
Cleveland, OH 44101
(800) 800-8661
$10.95 each

Self-healing audio tapes for: AIDS, asthma, arthritis, cancer, chemotherapy, depression, diabetes, high blood pressure/heart disease, and stroke.

Legal

It's in Your Hands (video tape)
Commission on Legal Problems of the Elderly
American Bar Association
1800 M Street, NW
Washington, DC 20036
(800) 237-4599
Videos may be rented for $18 or purchased for $48.

WillMaker (computer software)
Nolo Press
950 Parker Street
Berkeley, CA 94710
(510) 549-1976

Choice in Dying
250 W. 57th St.
New York, N.Y. 10107
Obtain free living will forms (send a self-addressed stamped envelope)

"Health Care Powers of Attorney"
Free brochure from the American Bar Association.
Send a postcard to:
AARP Fulfillment
No. D13895
P.O. Box 2110
Long Beach, CA 90801-2400
Power of attorney forms are available in some states from the state medical association, and at most hospitals and senior centers.

Travel

**Society for the Advancement of Travel
for the Handicapped**
347 5th Avenue, Suite 610
New York, NY 10016
(212) 447-7284

Chapter 14

Clothing, equipment and meals-by-mail, plus other useful items

---

Catalogues that specialize in aids for daily living:

Accessories for Daily Living
(800) 645-5272
Helpful and useful items.

Avenues Unlimited
(800) 848-2837
Clothing, accessories,workout videos and more for wheelchair users.

Comfortably Yours
(615) 867-9977
Various items to help with daily living.

Enrichments for Better Living
(800) 323-5547
Clothing and useful gadgets.

Extended Family
(800) 235-7070
Mail-order food service prepares 7 days worth of homemade, nutritious dinners and ships them anywhere in the country within two days. Free catalogue.

Feminine Image
(800) 576-3203
A catalogue featuring breast forms and other products for women who have had a mastectomy.

Healing Touches
(800) 576-3203
A catalogue featuring books, cosmetics, clothing and resources for information about breast cancer.

Homebound Resources, Ltd.
(512) 837-2777
Equipment, furniture and clothes.

Image Path
(800) 800-8661
Self-healing tapes for cancer.

IREP - Products Distributor
(800) 828-0852
Products for physical therapy and fitness.
Call for specific information and requests.

Fred Sammons' Catalog
(800) 323-554
Geriatric products.

Micro Bio-Medics, Inc.
(800) 241-6555
First-aid and athletic equipment, wheelchairs and rehabilitation equipment.

Products for the Physically Challenged
(800) 321-0595

Rifton Equipment
(800) 374-3866
Equipment for disabled children.

Sears Focus/Home Health Catalog
(800) 366-3000
Equipment and clothing.

Special Clothes
(703) 683-7343
Conventional-looking clothes for children size 2 toddler to 18 teen size.

Support Plus
(800) 229-2910
Hosiery, shoes and undergarments.

BIBLIOGRAPHY

Affairs in Order by Patricia Anderson

Before You Call the Doctor by Anne Simons, M.D., Bobbie Hasselbring, and Michael Castleman

Case Management by Nurses by Kathleen A. Bower, D.N.Sc., R.N.

How to Prepare for Death by Yaffa Draznin

It's Your Choice by Thomas C. Nelson

Kill as Few Patients as Possible by Oscar London, M.D.

On Death and Dying by Elisabeth Kubler-Ross

Parentcare Surival Guide by Enid Pritikin, M.S.W., L.C.S. W., and Trudy Reece, M.S.O.T.

Take This Book to the Hospital with You by Charles B. Inlander & Ed Weiner

Taking Care of Your Aging Famly Members by Nancy R. Hooyman and Wendy Lustbader

The Consumer's Legal Guide to Today's Health Care by Stephen L. Isaacs, J.D. and Ava C. Swartz, M.P.H.

When a Loved One is Ill by Leonard Felder, Ph.D.

You Don't Have to Suffer by Judy Tatelbaum

Your Aging Parents by John Deedy

INDEX

Order blank

To order *The Other Mid-Life Crisis: Everything You Need to Know About Wills, Hospitals, Life-and-Death Decisions and Final Matters (but were never taught)*, complete below and send with check to:
Meridian Publishing, Inc.
2431 Tulip Road,
San Jose, California 95128

Name _____

Street _____

City _____

State _____Zip _____

Please send me ___ copy (ies) of *The Other Mid-Life Crisis* at $14.95 each (add $2.00 per copy for shipping). Send check or money order (no cash). California residents please add 8 1/4% tax (.81¢ each book).

Total enclosed $_____
To order by credit card, call (800) 270-2116.
Bulk purchase inquiries invited.

-- *cut here* ---

To order *The Other Mid-Life Crisis: Everything You Need to Know About Wills, Hospitals, Life-and-Death Decisions and Final Matters (but were never taught)*, complete below and send with check to:
Meridian Publishing, Inc.
2431 Tulip Road,
San Jose, California 95128

Name _____

Street _____

City _____

State _____Zip _____

Please send me ___ copy (ies) of *The Other Mid-Life Crisis* at $14.95 each (add $2.00 per copy for shipping). Send check or money order (no cash). California residents please add 8 1/4% tax (.81¢ each book).

Total enclosed $_____
To order by credit card, call (800) 270-2116.
Bulk purchase inquiries invited.